Backwards

An Original Look from a Different Perspective

Cyndi Whatif

Purple Beaver Publishing
Alvin, Texas 77512

Health Backwards: An Original Look from a Different Perspective.

For information, contact Purple Beaver Publishing, PO Box 1114, Alvin, TX 77512 or contact@purplebeaverpublishing.com.

.

ISBN(s). Paperback: 979-8-9886104-0-3, eBook: 979-8-9886104-1-0, Hardback: 979-8-9886104-2-7

Library of Congress Number: 2023911770

First paperback edition August 2023

Foreword by Dr. Aaron Chapa, DC

Edited by Stuart Budgen, Michael Fedison

Cover art, infographics, and layout by Purple Beaver Publishing

Publisher's Cataloging-in-Publication data
Names: Whatif, Cyndi, author.
Title: Health backwards : an original look from a different perspective / Cyndi Whatif.
Description: Includes bibliographical references. | Alvin, TX: Purple Beaver Publishing, 2023.
Identifiers: LCCN: 2023911770 | ISBN: 979-8-9886104-2-7 (hardcover) | 979-8-9886104-0-3 (paperback) | 979-8-9886104-1-0 (ebook)
Subjects: LCSH Whatif, Cyndi. | Self-care, Health. | Holistic medicine. | Diseases--Alternative treatment. | Alternative medicine. | Allergy--Alternative treatment. | Inflammation--Alternative treatment. | BISAC
Health & Fitness/ Alternative Therapies | Health & Fitness/ Disease & Conditions / Chronic Fatigue | Health & Fitness/ Disease & Conditions/ Immune & Autoimmune | Health & Fitness/ Allergies | Health & Fitness/ Holism
Classification: LCC RA776 .W43 2023 | DDC 613--dc23

From me to you.

I see hope on the horizon.

Medical Disclaimer:

All content, media, and information contained in this book is for informational purposes ONLY.

I am sharing my personal experience. *It is NOT intended to be personal medical advice.* Only you and your doctor know your health.

Always seek professional medical advice. If you choose to act on any information in this book, you are doing so at your own risk.

This book should never be a substitute for professional medical advice from healthcare professionals. It is my personal experience.

Contents

Foreword

As a wellness doctor and lifestyle modification coach, I find great joy in accompanying people as they open up the vast door to taking responsibility for their health. Cyndi Wilson has done just that. She has studied her previous health challenges and understands the impact her family history has had on her wellbeing, but she has refused to allow it to define how she will finish her race.

The healthcare journey in today's world has become too focused on the goal of a quick-fix, Westernized pill. In reality, wellness should be a lifelong journey dedicated to staying healthy and maintaining the daily disciplines necessary to achieving that goal while educating others along the way.

Cyndi's journey to wellness is a great story demonstrating how, despite being exposed to so many life challenges, toxins, and harmful man-made substances, we can still find good health, vitality, and energy no matter how hopeless it can seem sometimes.

I am excited to see the impact Cyndi will make as she teaches others how to look at Health through a revolutionary new lens.

Dr. Aaron Chapa D.C.

Dr. Aaron Chapa is a Chiropractic Doctor who practices predominantly Clinical Nutrition. After graduating with honors from Texas Chiropractic College, he traveled all over the nation learning the leading applied kinesiology techniques with the top doctors in the country and utilizing the most advanced methods of drug-free healthcare.

He and his wife Tiffani began **Living Well Clinical Nutrition Center** in 2007. His practice revolves around the philosophy that the body wants to heal itself if given the right tools.

Introduction

"The best thing
a human being can do
is to help another
human being know more."
—Charlie Munger

INTRODUCTION

"I will be the first one to admit there is a lot of stuff I do not know; however, I do believe I know something everybody needs to know.

Opening Story: How it All Began

When I began the journey to put an end to my chronic fatigue, I saw "regular doctors" at first, but they had no viable answers for me. At one point, a doctor looked at me and said, "Why are we seeing you again?" I didn't look sick, I was in my ideal weight range most of the time, and they couldn't see *why* I needed help, let alone how to help me.

I was frustrated, but instead of giving up, I opted for alternative medicine. I was over forty years old when my naturopath diagnosed me with a pituitary gland problem that came with a life expectancy of thirty-eight to forty-two. I was devastated, so I did exactly what she recommended I do: I started taking human growth hormone shots four times a week. I had low blood pressure at the time, as well as an irregular heartbeat and a slew of other problems. I was even told I probably had multiple sclerosis (MS). I was only to proceed with the testing for MS if I was willing to take the medication for it.

My mom had been tested for MS when I was starting my freshman year in college. She had a bad reaction to the medication and ended up having many strokes. After two months of touch and go, she stabilized, but it took her two years before she was able to chew her food and another two years before she could finally say her first words again: "Hi, Doc." She never regained the use of her limbs on the right side of her body after that.

I was scared. I didn't want that for me, and since I was so allergic to everything, why would I not be allergic to the suggested medicine as well? I declined the test.

At this point, I had already spent years with acupuncturists and chiropractors, while using supplements, diet, and exercise. Nothing seemed to work. When I started getting tunnel vision on top of everything else, I was on the verge of accepting my fate. It was Christmas then. Would it be my last ever Christmas?

My husband and I shared our frustrations with a friend, and he recommended we give a homeopathic practitioner he knew a try before resorting to MS diagnosis and medication. I was tired of trying. Tired of hoping. I thought homeopaths were only placebos for people who needed someone to take their hand and say, "There, there." Had I really fallen this low? But I didn't have any other options left. *Sigh.*

I went to see her. I was too weak to drive, so my husband took me. On the way there, he looked over at me and said, "If she pulls out a crystal ball, we are leaving." (We don't know what we don't know, I guess.)

We had no idea what to expect. She said she was able to help me. However, since we were at the opposite ends of the spectrum with our spiritual beliefs, I felt compelled to research everything she suggested before doing it. I had so many questions, and she was very accommodating. I ended up doing everything she told me to do. I became fully functional again after about nine months. I had to avoid so many things though... and on top of that, I was only allowed to eat about ten specific foods in all.

I had to keep so many plates spinning during that time. I felt like I was a ticking time bomb. With six kids—one being only two years old at the time—I continued going to see her for another two years, until all the plates finally came crashing down around me. It was at this point my husband refused to let me see her anymore. I went on medication for one month. It was a bad month. Alternative medicine couldn't help me, Western medicine couldn't help me, so I was all alone. But I'm not a quitter, and I decided to put my Bachelor of Science brain to use and figure this out by myself.

I'm now 54 years old as I'm writing this. I have cured myself of all previously mentioned health issues. I'm not saying all my health issues are gone, but I'm slowly notching them off one at a time. I spent hundreds of hours learning and gathering the information I'm going to share here. I filled over fifteen notebooks full to be more precise. I'm only going to sum up the highlights though, so I can keep it as short as possible. There is a lot of information, but it all boils down to a very simple concept at its core. However, implementing all of it can be quite tricky, but not impossible given the proper guidelines.

It makes me think of the meme I saw about learning how to play bass guitar. In this meme there is a thin notebook that says, *How to Play Bass Guitar*. Next to it is a towering book 1,000 times thicker that says, *How to Play Bass Guitar Well.* That's kind of like what I'm sharing in this book: the simple basics or the thin book—even though it's still a bit thick.

Please understand I'm trying to share the foundation of a whole new concept, so there is a significant amount of material to cover. If you take it in small bites, hopefully it will not be too overwhelming.

When I was trapped in this learning process, sometimes I wished I hadn't figured out what I'd discovered. Like in the popular movie *The Matrix*, when Neo needed to decide if he wanted to know the truth, and Morpheus tells him once he is told it, he can never go back. Well, that's exactly what it was like for me. I knew there was a problem, but the problem was hidden. In the beginning when I was figuring this out, I felt just like Neo—depressed, scared, alone, wishing I didn't know—but at the same time I was glad I did. Glad I was able to live fourteen years (so far) past the expiration date my doctor gave me. You see, I had been putting up with over a decade of being told my health problems were all in my head. Now they were telling me they weren't. So, when I was actually told about my life expectancy, I was not shocked. What could I do about it though? Nothing? What would you do?

Though everyone looked at Neo as The Chosen One who would fix everything, I certainly wasn't. I think my family and doctors looked at me as a feeble creature who fell off the deep end with her diagnosis. What it really was, though, was sheer frustration and hopelessness. I had been living a healthy lifestyle for decades. It didn't work. Not only did it not work, but it also brought me to this point. I figured, what do I have to lose? I'm already living on borrowed time. I must go down fighting.

Strangely enough though, I stayed alive. In fact, not only did I stay alive, but I started feeling better than I ever had. Of course, this did cause me to be a little nervous about proceeding down this road alone. I now felt like I was living instead of just putting in my time. I now had something to lose. I was no longer being forced to choose between jumping off the steep cliff into the river below or being shot. It's scarier to jump when you're not forced to. I jumped anyway, and I kept going. I didn't want to go backward and have all those symptoms return. It wasn't an option.

Like Neo, I survived, and I grew in knowledge and confidence. At some point, I did eventually break the code to my health *Matrix*. All of the pieces fell into place, and it all finally made sense. Well, at least to me it did. But the problem here is I still needed help. I still needed to be fixed. Just because I understood the problem didn't make the problem go away. I knew there were people who had far more information about the human body and what it needed than I did, but at least now what they did recommend could be manipulated in a way I could actually benefit from. Because of this, I needed someone else to understand my predicament too. Like the Matrix uploads, my health care professional and I needed to be running on the same program in order for proper communication to happen. I needed their help but... there was still a communication barrier.

In the process of trying to explain to them what I had figured out, I continued to learn more. I knew I had only scraped the tip of the iceberg, and the tentacles appeared to reach further than I ever imagined. But the deeper down the rabbit hole I went, the more I noticed it always led to the same field I am about to share here.

My hope in writing this book is to have both sides of the medical world rethink what they know. To see how they can actually work together to help us with our health. I hope there will emerge an expert for each specific rabbit hole. I hope they will evaluate what they already know in light of this new information. I know what I discovered worked for me, but I need help finding out if it's possible for it to be true for others as well.

Looking from a Different Angle

"Future medicine will be the medicine of frequencies."

—Albert Einstein

How can this be? **If Einstein is correct, does it also mean the future of illnesses will be related to frequencies as well?** Is this why we have so many invisible illnesses? Are we looking for something, we can't actually see?

Your first reaction may be, "No, invisible illnesses are predominantly autoimmune diseases that cannot be seen. We look healthy but are not." Touché. But *what if* the genesis of the inflammation that causes the symptoms to autoimmune diseases was because of frequencies? What if undiagnosed health challenges were occurring for the same reason?

When I was looking for a way to fix my health problems, some of which probably stemmed from Camp Lejeune water poisoning,[1] I discovered a missing body system. When I understood the details of how this system worked, I was able to eliminate my inflammation regularly. If symptoms from inflammation are the cause of the many discomforts with autoimmune disease, could removing the inflammation correct the problem?

In this book, I am going to speculate on the physical side of energy healing. My view is not spiritual in nature, nor is it chakra related. I don't know anything about those techniques. I give those a wide berth. However, I do have a hypothesis I have developed over the past decade. Acting on this hypothesis eliminated my environmental sensitivities and my high intolerance to many foods. When I implemented it, inflammation stopped within hours. It worked consistently for me when doctors could not find a way to help me.

If you have picked this book up to find the secret to curing your health challenges, I'm sorry, but I cannot say *use this or take that and you will be well*. It is more than that. It is bigger than that. It's more like trying to learn how to fly without realizing there is such a thing as gravity. We can't see gravity. We had to accept the possibility that maybe there was something going on we could not see. We can only see how gravity acts on other objects. However, the more we studied gravity, the more we learned about it, and the more we could work around it to accomplish what we wanted—flight. Refusing to believe gravity existed definitely would not make it easier to get off the ground. But accepting the idea that

---

[1] Freshwater, Lori Lou. "What Happened at Camp Lejeune." *psmag*, Grist, 21 August 2018.

maybe something was keeping us bound to the earth could give us a way to work around it to accomplish our goal—which we obviously did.

I believe what I have stumbled across is like gravity. It is something invisible that affects our health immensely, and it may never actually be seen by the human eye. When I gave the benefit of the doubt that this invisible system did exist, things happened. Progress was made. Progress I could not achieve previously when following a healthy lifestyle, nor taking medication. Does this make it the missing key for other health challenges? Maybe. I definitely think it is the missing key to inflammation and nutritional deficiencies.

This *new gravity*, so to speak, is what I want to reveal in this book. For healthy people, this invisible system works properly. For unhealthy people, this system malfunctioning causes the body to appear to turn on itself (inflammation). I believe what the body is really doing is trying to protect us from hurting ourselves more. I believe inflammation is a sign that this hidden system is malfunctioning. This inflammation creates a chain reaction. I believe this chain reaction causes nutrient and hormone imbalances. So many health challenges today are caused by these two things—inflammation and nutritional deficiencies. With these two problems gone, how much less health problems would there be?

What the Reader Can Expect to Gain

At this point of the book, I could bore you with all of the statistics out there focusing on these specific health problems. I could tell you how barely five percent of the population lives symptom free.[2] Or how sixty percent of American adults have at least one chronic condition while forty-two percent have more than one.[3] I think we are all well aware of this already. I am here to say I do believe these problems are there. I do believe that, in spite of the efforts taken to prevent it, lives are still lost. A lot of lives. I believe we need to remember they are real people, not just numbers.

I also believe that when I felt helpless and was told there was no known cure, I wanted these feelings to go away at any cost, but what could I do? I was already doing what was *supposed* to work and it wasn't working. I decided even if it was just the act of doing something—anything, even if it was the unusual—if it could remove these heart-wrenching feelings of helplessness... I would do it. So, I did. I was willing to accept the possibility—or even the probability—that no progress would be made, but I still thought it was worth a try. I could say I did my best.

If it wasn't for my kids, I probably would have given up on the fight to survive. I had started hearing about the reports coming out about Camp Lejeune water poisoning. It was very possible my health problems stemmed from this catastrophe. My mom had become pregnant with me after living there for

---

[2] Rettner, Rachael. "Are You the 5 Percent? Small Minority Have No Health Problems." LiveScience. 7 June 2015. https://www.livescience.com/51122-world-health-problems.html.

[3] Irving, Doug. "Chronic Conditions in America: Price and Prevalence." *Rand Corporation* (blog). 12 July 2017. https://www.rand.org/blog/rand-review/2017/07/chronic-conditions-in-america-price-and-prevalence.html.

a few years. This was the legacy I was going to leave my kids? My drive became intense. If it was too late for me, maybe I could figure something out for them. Something to prevent them from having to carry this burden.

I know, why me? Well, why not me? If you have ever read the book *Blink* by Malcolm Gladwell, it talks about how sometimes the less a person knows, the easier it is to see what is really happening.

Don't get me wrong, I had gone to college and earned a Bachelor of Science. I had also been averaging a book a month, cover to cover, for years, trying to find the elusive next thing to avoid this 'health hellhole' I had witnessed my mom, dad, sisters, and nephews fall into. But it didn't make any difference. Why? Why wasn't what was *supposed to work* working?

For example, statistics tell us the number of people dying, the number of people infected, and the number of people vaccinated for COVID-19. Even though vaccinations have been around for centuries, the only disease considered to be eradicated by this method is smallpox—and it took more than just vaccinations in order for it to happen.[4] COVID is still here. We are told to get booster after booster, but it's still not working. Is this what the world is going to be like for the next century? God, I hope not. But I say what fools we are to think

---

[4] World Health Organization. "Smallpox Eradication Program—SEP (1966–1980)." World Health Organization. 1 May 2010. https://www.who.int/news-room/feature-stories/detail/the-smallpox-eradication-programme---sep-(1966-1980).

the old way of just vaccinating is going to fix everything. It hasn't fixed anything yet.

What if we needed to look at this problem from a totally different angle?

What if we just grouped COVID with all the other health problems and looked for the most common denominators among them? What if we proceeded from there, but ***BACKWARDS***?

How This Book is Organized

I have broken this book down into seven sections. Each section and chapter builds upon the previous one. To get the most out of the book, I strongly encourage you to read it in order.

The Book Is Arranged as Follows:

1. Introduction: Getting in the Correct Mindset
2. Laying the Groundwork: Chapters 1–3
3. Understanding the System: Chapters 4–6
4. Working the System: Chapters 5–9
5. Magnitude of DISH: Chapters 10–12
6. Conclusion: Key Takeaways
7. More Information: Glossary and Appendices

Each chapter begins with a glimpse of my personal experience which leads to the information in the chapter. I share the information I learned using three main points and give examples of how the information was used and what happened as a result of it. For the first half of the book, I share the different perspective I have found and give thought-provoking questions for you to consider. In the second half of the book, I dive into what I have learned about this new concept and end each chapter with a summary of the steps I took.

Keep in mind, I am trying to condense ten years of learning into a manageable book. This book is intended to give you an overview of a possible system in the body we didn't know previously existed. I will use the simple parts of a machine to illustrate this concept. I have left out all the small moving parts. It is the freshly cut jungle trail.

One last quick note on how I wrote this book. Forgive me if I sound too elementary, but I prefer to keep things simple. I will be using my own simple vocabulary and many analogies.

✓ I use analogies because they make it easier to grasp new concepts.

✓ I have designated the main analogies with colored arrows.

✓ The most frequently used new vocabulary words are these four:

- **Good Guys:** Anything the body should have in it.

  vitamins, minerals, amino acids, hormones, etc.

- **Bad Guys:** Anything the body should NOT have in it.

  viruses, bacteria, parasites, radiation, chemicals, etc.

- **Shield:** This is what makes the mystery system possible.

- **DISH:** Defensive Individual *Shield* Hypothesis.

  What I believe is the hidden piece to the puzzling questions about our health challenges.

There are several other words I've adapted or created to explain this mystery system. I will introduce them gradually. I have also included a glossary at the end of the book.

How to Use This Book

Please remember, this is not a how-to manual. It is a what-I-did narrative. It is intended for the reader to look at a subject from a different perspective knowing full well in advance it is a very new concept. A concept that worked for me, but only by glancing backward as I proceeded forward. A concept that, if accurate, should work for others, but with far too many factors for me to be able to give any detailed advice about. It is a lonely road. I would never have even found the trailhead if I hadn't already been told what areas of my body had problems (medical doctor), what deficiencies my body was experiencing (naturopath doctor), and the factors that were affecting me (homeopathic doctor).

This book does not answer specific questions for specific illnesses. It is more like a formula for the math problem so the problem can be solved for multiple situations. It is a simple concept, but implementing it is difficult. It is like the difference between using a calculator or manually doing a long division problem like 252,815 divided by 857. Not easy manually, but doable—whereas the same problem can be done very quickly with a calculator. Both would produce the same answer. When this body system is functioning properly, it is like using a calculator. When it is not, it is pen and paper and the many guesses required to solve the long division problem. It still works but takes more time and thought in order to arrive at the answer of 295.

Sometimes just coming up with the correct questions can be the hardest part.

I originally planned to share only the simple side of the answer in this book, but as I was seeking feedback, I was asked to provide more details. They wanted me to go deeper and tell them more. I did do this, which is why the book has so many pages. I am going to lay out the entire math formula for you. This does not mean I am suggesting you run off and do it. I would suggest you find a health practitioner who is open to the idea of this formula and will help you plug in the factors needed. I used this formula with the factors my health professionals gave me. Doing this enabled what previously didn't work for me to now work.

I would recommend you read this book and decide for yourself if you think this may be something you and your healthcare professional should discuss.

What I Hope for the Reader

My desire is that I give you hope. I know, sometimes hope is cruel. I'm sorry. But hope we must. These days, we are continually being informed by Fact Checkers that something has not been proven or confirmed by a reliable source. How about instead of relying on Fact Checkers, we check it out ourselves?

Maybe... We Don't Know What We Don't Know.

Or... We Don't Know What We Do Know.

As you read, I ask you to set aside what you already know and ask yourself if this new perspective logically makes sense. I don't go into any advanced science. It is basically math and science concepts most of us learned in junior high. If we are fact-checking the broad assumptions and disregarding anything contrary to them, we may be preventing ourselves from moving forward.

"Rarely are we lucky enough to have to make such dramatic changes in our assumptions that a really major breakthrough becomes possible."[5]

What if... we take the famous philosopher, René Descartes' advice? Let's go back to square one. Begin from the very minimal of assumptions instead of from what we already know. This quote from *The Story of Philosophy* by Bryan Magee summarizes perfectly what Descartes thought.

> *I found that in moving only by logical steps, each of which was simple and obvious, from premises each of which was also simple and obvious, you began to reach conclusions that were not at all simple and not at all obvious.*[6]

---

[5] Roberts, Richard J. "Ten Simple Rules to Win a Nobel Prize." *PLOS Computational Biology*. 2 April 2015. https://journals.plos.org/ploscompbiol/article?id=10.1371/journal.pcbi.1004084.

[6] Magee, Bryan. *The Story of Philosophy* (A Dorling Kindersley Book, 1998), 86.

What if... going back further to square one led down a different path, causing many rabbit holes to show up in the same field?

What if... it made all medical approaches work better and caused a turnaround in the national health care crisis?

What would happen if we started back with only the known fact of like waves canceled—destructive interference?

Where would it lead science? It led me to writing this book.

Section 1

Thought Process to This Different Perspective

CHAPTER 1:

SEEING WHAT CAN'T BE SEEN

We are missing something, and it may never be seeable; however, it does not make it unfindable.

Opening Story: Living in a Tent

Once upon a time, I was told some joke or stupid phrase where the ending went something like, "The crazy person is the only one who doesn't know he is crazy." I can't count how many times those words circulated through my mind, or how many times caring people would gently hint at this. Talk about a stab to the heart. I must believe they were well meaning, but it didn't take away the pain. Though I felt like I was the only one going through unexplainable health challenges, I knew I wasn't.

During one of my last trips to the small gym I frequented, I met a lady in the locker room. When I had walked into the changing area, she started apologizing profusely for the smell she had created. The only thing she could safely clean her body with was apple cider vinegar of all things. We got to talking. We unfortunately had so much in common. She lived in a tent on her front porch out in the country. She knew her beautiful home made her sick. She went on to say that even being there in the gym, she was starting to feel her allergic reactions come on. She came here to shower and leave as fast as she could because her husband would get mad when she smelled up their house.

At the time, I knew I couldn't handle computer or television screens. At one point, if these devices were active on the same level of the house as I was on (it was a two-story) I would immediately feel dizzy, nauseous, and have stomach pain. Easy enough: we just didn't turn them on. We continually cut things out of our life, just to get by. A little before it got to this point, I used to stand in the doorway and give instructions to my teenage daughter on what I would want her to look up online for me. I would have her print out any potential interesting data I could read later to help me try to figure out what was wrong with me. I could usually only do this for ten to twenty minutes unless I was sitting. I would then be able to make it to thirty minutes.

Later, I came to find out two of my sisters would not use electricity in their houses. They would use a wood stove to cook. They said they felt so much better since doing so. *Yeah, but you sound like a freak...*

Not long after, I reluctantly joined their freak club. I was symptom free and had energy... if I was outside. We lived out in the country. When people pulled up our driveway, they saw tents—one for the girls and one for my young boys. They saw a picnic table and a makeshift stove. They saw my kids running around having a blast while I sat in my lawn chair reading the pages I'd had my daughter print out for me earlier. They thought I was a thoughtful mom with the kids' interest at heart. No, I was just rejoicing that I could think and not be in pain. I had to be out there. The kids wanted to be out there too. So, I let them. We did this for over a month.

At night, the sadness would come. I would go inside long enough to prepare for bed and then, as my husband would go to his bed, I would head out to my tent. My three-year-old daughter at the time thought it was fun to get to sleep outside with Mom every night. We would sit by the candlelight, and she would talk nonstop. She would get all the words out of her head for the day. Her older siblings wouldn't be around to interrupt her or complete her sentences for her. After an hour, I would just say, "Okay, time to stop talking and go to sleep now."

"Okay, night Mom." And that was it.

I knew the days were getting shorter, and the autumn storms would come and I would have to go back inside. I still could not prove at this point that it was the electricity affecting me. I was still being accused of it being mental. How was it possible to be almost symptom free outside the house when I was affected so badly inside? And why was nobody else? Was it the house's building materials? Was it really the electricity? Was I just really crazy? Or what?

It came: the first storm of the year. The tents were not going to be able to withstand it. My husband insisted everyone come inside. We had to lower the tents so they wouldn't blow away. I sat wrapped in a blanket on the tiny steps of the back porch under the awning as long as I could. His tone of voice told me he was annoyed at me. That I was being ridiculous. I would agree with him. But, but...

When the awning stopped providing protection against the horizontal wind and rain, I had no choice. I went inside. Within ten minutes, my whole body felt like how I imagined a locust must feel when he needed to shed his shell for a larger size. Pressure everywhere. My body trapped. The feeling of well-being quickly escaped my body. How could I get him to understand something was not right physically?

Boom. Flicker. The power went out. My body sighed in relief. I felt fine again. For four hours, I felt like I was outside. I went about by candlelight doing the severely neglected chores. It made me realize, no matter how much everyone else thought it was in my head, I knew something I could not see was preventing me from having a normal life. I also learned that, once the power was back on, having the switches off in the room was not enough. The low frequency flowing through the walls was still affecting me. However, cutting the electricity breaker in the room I was in did work. I didn't need to look for a winter tent. I could be inside! I just needed to stay predominantly in the family room. It was where we cut the power.

Since I am writing this book on my computer, in my house, I am obviously not like this anymore. I am no longer in survival mode only. Why is that? Well, it wasn't because of a particular diet, medication, or even psychiatric help. It was because of something I very slowly figured out over time. Part of me wants to just leave the past behind because I no longer live in daily desperation, and I definitely don't want to dwell there in my mind either, but this is the selfish side of me. The side that is telling me to hide; trying so hard to quiet my big sister's voice in my head: "Nobody cares to hear what you have to say."

I remember the lady in the gym. I met someone waiting outside for her doctor's appointment because being inside the building made her feel like throwing up from all the smells. I remember my sister who cooks over a wood stove not to be economical, but to feel less symptomatic. I feel sorry for them. I feel selfish if I just stop at feeling sorry for them. I know everyone is different; everyone is unique. But I also know most people have eyeballs on their faces and not their buttocks. What if what I figured out worked for others? I at least have to share and let them decide for themselves. Let them at least have hope that maybe something invisible is the problem. And though many will say it is electricity, it may not be. But it may be just as invisible.

We know the lymphatic system and the immune system are closely connected. We associate a strong immune system with the lymphatic system doing its job. The job we can see through a microscope. We can visually see what I will call Security Guards. These Security Guards would roam around looking for trouble, i.e., Bad Guys. If these Security Guards would come across Bad Guys, they would send out a special detachment of Attackers to get rid of them. This method has a very efficient way of doing the needed job. But, for some of us, not so much. These Attacker characters might decide the Bad Guys are too much work and just let them go. Or these Attackers could get carried away and go nuts, not caring if Good Guys were affected too.

Why is that?

What if something else was going on? Something we cannot see under a microscope.

What if it is about not only what they *are* doing but what they *aren't* doing as well?

If we need to rely on the immune system to get well, and the immune system is already doing all it can (or, worse yet, doing more than it should in the case of autoimmune disease), is there something that can be done besides what is already being done? Instead of only looking at what is being done, let us look at what is not being done as well.

What if this lymphatic system was responsible for the creation of a different system we didn't even know was there? What if this system complemented the immune system and was the determining factor in how effective the immune system could be? Maybe this mystery system is doing something for us we aren't aware of yet.

I think this system working determines whether or not a person has the opportunity to be healthy.

For me, figuring out this mystery system at least gave my body the chance to do what it was supposed to be doing. How? I started manually doing what this system is supposed to be doing automatically until it was able to do it on its own again. I guess you could say it was like priming the pump of a dried-up old-fashioned water spigot. Pump it enough times manually and the water would eventually start flowing freely.

The New Perspective

What it all boiled down to for me was this complementary mystery system. Not only did I stumble across this system, but through much blood, sweat, tears, research, and prayer, I learned how to manually do this complementary system's job until my body was finally able to handle the load without assistance.

Now it's time for our first big analogy.

Bike Analogy

What I came to discover was that, for me, this complementary system went wrong in two ways. I guess the best way to describe it is to look at the body like it's a bicycle. It doesn't matter if the tires are aired up, the rims are not bent, the seat height is good, the pedals are not broken, and so on. **If the chain was broken, I wasn't going anywhere.** I think this might be why so many tests came back negative for me.

What Is the Chain?

I think the chain is a "sorting system" the body is supposed to automatically be doing. I figured out how to get the chain back on! I figured out how to get my body to start sorting again. In the beginning, the chain still fell off a lot. But as I understood it more, I was able to fine-tune the gears.

The more fine-tuning I did, the less often the chain fell off the gears. Now, my sorting system is working more often than not. My chain is now on the gears more than off the gears.

With the chain staying on the gears, I have high hopes of being able to someday bike across the finish line! How did I make this sorting system work? I focused on the chain, not the bike. I focused on a three-step process.

A) The chain was broken: Something broke my chain.

Something caused my body to stop "sorting" and clearing Bad Guys efficiently. There was probably a physical reason for this—the trigger—but because it stayed this way for so long, something else happened as well. I suspected it was a type of "disconnect," and because of this disconnect, I needed to retrain my brain to remind my body what to do.

We know involuntary actions like blinking can also be voluntary. What about other functions of the body? It was worth a shot, and it worked! But it wasn't enough for me. For some, this may be enough. This may be why the thinking-yourself-healthy approach works for many. This may also be why it doesn't work for all people.

B) Fix the chain: This was putting missing information back into my brain.

I noticed my brain didn't like missing data. My brain needed to know how things I encountered in my environment on a regular basis connected to similar objects in my past. My subconscious brain could not remember on its own. It was like the road was blocked and it was looking for a detour to take to get where it needed to be. Helping the brain to remember these connections was fixing the chain. I would need to consciously think about how things were associated with each other. Doing this would somehow "kick-start" the subconscious mind to know how to process whatever it was it needed to process. Was this neuroplasticity taking place? Neuroplasticity, generally speaking, is when one part of the brain takes over the job of an injured part of the brain. Or... was I re-creating pathways in the brain? Or both? I didn't know. I do know it was working. So, I kept doing it. However, fixing the chain wasn't enough.

C) Put the chain back on the gears: I manually did the sorting system's job.

I did this by getting to know my body through muscle testing—also called sway testing. I wanted to understand what my body was trying to tell me. I started altering my surroundings deliberately in what I call batches. I made my allergies work for me and not against me. If you have had any chronic illness for any period of time, you probably already know what it is like to need certain routines or schedules in order to make it through the day. It is like this but with progress forward! With lasting change! I have named this missing system Defensive Individual Shield Hypothesis (DISH). The concept is simple; implementing it is a different story.

Getting Started

Throughout the book I will be giving examples of my experiences. These examples are not meant as medical advice. They are to help you visualize the concept I am explaining. They are meant to encourage you to think in a broader sense. To start asking questions. New questions. Questions that may, Lord willing, lead down a different road instead of always ending up at a dead end.

Taped across the bottom of my computer screen, I have a quote from an unknown source: "Tell the story of the mountain you climbed. Your words could be a page in someone else's survival guide." This is the quote that has pushed me past the fear of writing this book. The book that may very well be in the hands of a person who is stranded on the Island of Poor Health with No Answer Lagoon surrounding her. I will not say this book is the only way to get off this godforsaken island, but I can say it is what I used to get free. I wish I could promise more, but I can't. This is my own journey. If I just say, "May you have safe travels," it feels so heartless. But if I say there are several books out there that might help, and this just may be one of them, I can live with that regardless if you accept this information or not. I did my part.

There may always be a gap in the medical field some of us will fall through. I aim to make the gap smaller. I know my health is ultimately up to me. I can't shove my doctor in my pocket and bring him home to help me day to day. I needed to figure out a way to make what was supposed to work, work for me.

Thought to Ponder

As my kids were studying the Oregon Trail, they could not believe how people thought nothing about drinking water that contained floaties in it. Of course, this was coming from children who couldn't even stand drinking the pulp of orange juice. Well, those early frontier folks not only had no choice, but some of them didn't really see the significance of floaties affecting their health. Why? Because water that looked clear and harmless was sometimes more deadly (cholera bacterium). They could not see what was there. It also took twelve hours to five days for the symptoms to show up.[7]

Back in the 1600s, two centuries before the Oregon Trail time period, a Dutch amateur scientist named Antonie Philips van Leeuwenhoek played around with making lenses. He ended up making the first microscope. He showed his invention to the Royal Society in London. They were impressed and elected him to become a member. One day,

---

[7] Centers for Disease Control and Prevention. "Cholera—Vibrio cholerae infection." Centers for Disease Control and Prevention. 30 September 2022. https://www.cdc.gov/cholera/general/index.html.

he was experimenting with his invention and decided to focus on a drop of water. What he found he called wretched beasties. He shared his findings with the members of the Royal Society. None of them thought to make the connection between what they were looking at and the contagium that caused the Black Plague.[8]

Not too much thought was given to these wretched beasties until Louis Pasteur came onto the scene. He saw what everyone else saw but he realized there was relevance to it. From his diligent searching, he learned about yeast being alive and growing. He learned about bacteria and how germs contributed to health problems.

Are we seeing something relevant without realizing it when we look at energy fields around people? We have been observing them for centuries if you include Chinese acupuncture. Since we don't totally understand them, we throw it aside as pseudoscience or spiritual gobbledygook. I'm guilty. I thought so. However, I came to find out the relevance of this energy field as it pertained to my health. It is no longer magical or mystical to me. It turns out to be helpful and explainable with basic science learned in junior high.

Conclusion for Chapter 1

The natural thing to want to do is to give a name to what our health challenges are. "I have ______" (fill in the blank). Like this is supposed to summarize everything that is wrong. We want friends and family to understand our struggle. We want

---

[8] Dietz, David. *All About Great Medical Discoveries* (Random House, 1960), 36.

them to understand we are doing the best we can. But how do I do that when the problem isn't found? Besides, being able to pin it down doesn't necessarily help. As you will see as my story unfolds: it didn't help me.

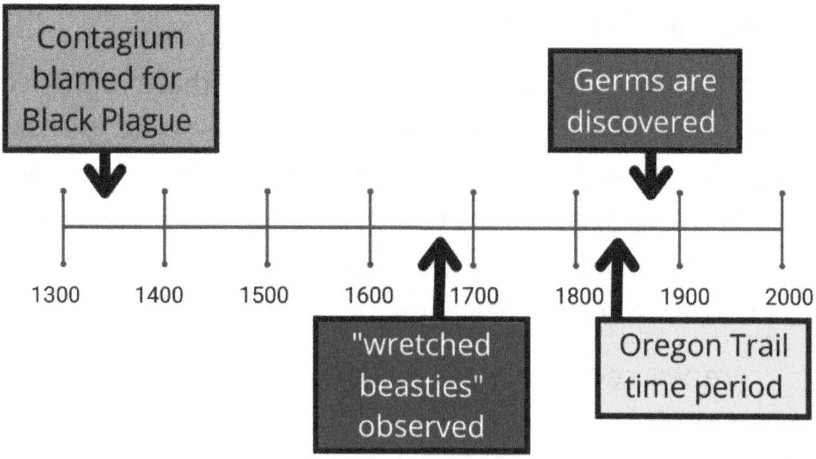

Yes, there was something wrong, but instead of finding a name and moving on, I wanted *it* fixed. To fix *it*, I had to know what *it* was. What was causing my health problems? Not the Bad Guy, but what in my body wasn't working?

I now believe *it* is the complementary mystery system malfunctioning. I believe this malfunctioning caused two problems. Two fixable problems. Not easy, but doable.

In summary:

As I mentioned before, I have named the proposed shield around our bodies the Defensive Individual Shield Hypothesis (DISH). If DISH is working, I can be healthy. If DISH is not working, I don't have an opportunity to improve my health. The reason being that the broken DISH causes missing information and misinformation.

- The problem is misinformation and missing information.
    - Misinformation caused deficiencies in my body.
    - Deficiencies caused missing information to happen.
    - Missing information prevented my body from functioning properly.
- The solution is to correct the problem.
    - Stop the misinformation from occurring.
    - Replenish the deficiencies.
    - Insert the missing information.
    - Avoid misinformation from happening again.

The solution is not easy, but it is doable.

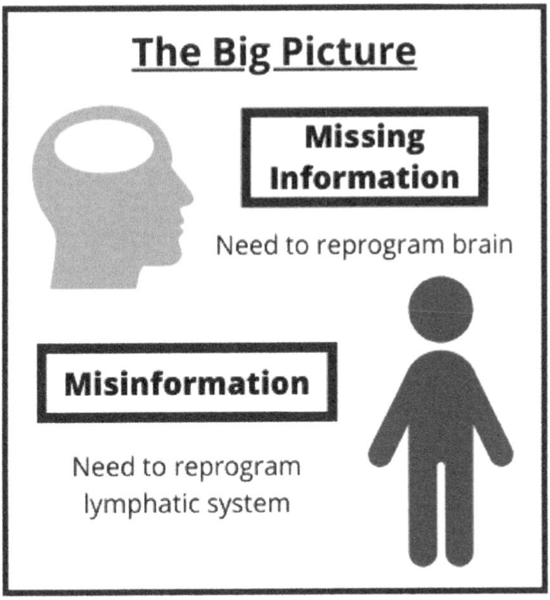

CHAPTER 2: BACK TO SQUARE ONE

If we keep going down the same path,

we will keep getting the same results.

Opening Story: Total Body Fast Did Not Work

I had heard of how doing a total body fast for 4 to 10 days could help my body to reset. I went down the road again of thinking maybe this was the one thing I was missing. I didn't want to try it, but I felt I had no choice. I was having unexplainable symptoms I could not turn on and off at cue for the doctors to observe, so how could they help? I was allergic to so much food at this point even though I was trying to be so careful. Any time I tried to eat anything, I would experience what my mom used to tell me she would experience. My throat would get tight and I could feel foam building up in my throat to where I could not swallow or breathe properly.

I guess eating was to be added to the things my body would no longer allow me to do. How does one survive without eating? My frustration and fear of eating my food was really making me *hangry.* Knowing that negative emotions on top of everything else would only add more complications (so I am told) I didn't want to go down that road also, right?

I ended up doing a water fast for 20 days. Coming out of this fast revealed three things:

1. I didn't lose or gain a single pound.

I reiterate, 20 days. I would say impossible. According to the Mifflin-St Jeor equation, I should have been burning at least 1,178 calories a day.[9] It takes 3,500 calories to burn one pound.[10] If I wasn't taking any in, I should have lost six-plus pounds over this period. But I didn't. I didn't even lose half a pound. The math did not add up correctly. Confusion.

2. Did the reset work? Yes and no.

Yes, because I was eventually able to eat very limited amounts. One item at a time. However, I was no better off. Nothing was different or better than the week before my hospital stay.

3. I found a hidden boldness deep inside of me that came spewing out.

I knew something was off. I knew it was not in my head. I knew the methods available were not working and would not work. I knew I was missing something. (This was before I knew about the Camp Lejeune water contamination.) I became resolved to figuring it out, and I didn't care if I died trying.

---

[9] Peele, Leigh. Writer & Information Digger. "Mifflin St. Jeor Calculator." Leigh Peele. Date unknown. https://www.leighpeele.com/mifflin-st-jeor-calculator.

[10] Johnson, Jolie. "How to Equate One Pound to Calories Burned & Carbs Burned." Live Strong. Last accessed 23 March 2023. https://www.livestrong.com/article/191454-how-to-equate-one-pound-to-calories-burned-carbs-burned/.

Overview

We only know what we know from what we have experienced or have been told. Sometimes, going back to the beginning and starting over results in going down the same path again and again without any change. We don't know of any other way. I'm from a large family. All of my siblings and parents had health challenges. They frequented the doctor and did as they were told, and they were no better off than me. In fact, I would venture to say, they were a little worse off. I guess I could say I decided to be the variable. I was going to try something different. I didn't want to end up where they were.

My something different was being a health nut. The key, or so we are told, to good health. This was not the key for me. Many years of trying and pushing through chronic fatigue, trying health key after health key, I had admitted defeat. None of those keys worked on unlocking my door to good health. Okay, then what? When I don't even know where to begin, it is overwhelming. Over time, I would meet people who had used different approaches to health. They seemed weird to me and I seemed weird to them. It's funny how whatever our normal is, we think is normal for everyone. So what *is* normal?

Normal is being faced with an obstacle and having to make a decision based on prior experience to anticipate the best decision. Everyone's choice would be different. Mine was to start digging. Start researching. Start looking for another path. When I hit bottom and had nothing to lose, I could either give up or get determined. I became determined. Determined to find out why, in spite of everything I was doing, I was still unable to embrace normal life activities without health ramifications.

I know some people just fall through the gap. They can't be helped. But could this gap be made smaller? Could I pull myself up out of this gap? Could I prevent my kids from falling into it? I had to try. I decided to go back to the beginning, and to assume as little as possible.

Topic 1: Trying to Think Differently is So Hard

Being Open-Minded

For 1,400 years, everybody thought the earth stood still—1,400 years! (That is a LONG TIME.) Copernicus saw it differently. He pointed out how a person on a ship could not tell he was moving based on his observation of the other objects on the ship with him. But when observing the shore, he could tell the ship was moving.[11]

He suggested this was the same for the earth. The sun didn't revolve around the earth, but the earth revolved around the sun. He looked at the situation from a different angle. He looked at it backwards. He wasn't disagreeing with everything else learned about outer space. In fact, all the information already known about the universe made even more sense when looked at from his angle.

That is all I am suggesting here. Let's look at what we know about health and our body from a different angle. But paradigm shifts are so difficult. We are told and henceforth believe what we are told for so long that to think there is any other way is a huge challenge. It has to be a deliberate decision.

My first deliberate decision was to give alternative medicine a chance. This path to alternative medicine was very slow for me. I wasn't stubborn. I was just suspicious. Even so, situations would continually be put in my path that would

---

[11] Ball, R. S. *Great Astronomers* (Kessinger Publishing, Date unknown), 19.

slowly point me in this new direction. I've heard it said the only reason these new techniques worked was because I had to believe they did. Not true for me. I was as skeptical as they come.

I know modern medicine is amazing. I wouldn't want to live life without it. I also know it was missing something. But I didn't even know where to look besides the standard protocol of diet, exercise, avoid harmful habits, and the like. I finally realized there may be more to "that other stuff" than meets the eye when I was getting a complimentary leg and foot massage after I had a caesarean delivery. It was standard protocol at this hospital. I thought, *Interesting. If a hospital warrants this as* standard protocol*, is there more to a massage than just a spa treatment?*

As the masseuse was massaging my left foot, she asked me if I had been having trouble with my right shoulder. Yes! I almost couldn't use my right arm for my last trimester. How could she know about my right shoulder pain by rubbing my left foot?

This led me to being open-minded about the effectiveness of acupuncture, which, in spite of the foot massage experience, I was still reluctant to try. I went, and, to be honest, I don't know if I would have gone back if I didn't feel any results after my first treatment. Evidently, it sometimes takes several treatments before any results are felt. Not for me. The following day my chronic fatigue was gone. For several years it stayed gone with periodic appointments. But things were still not correct with my body. I will leave it at that. I don't want to TMI (too much information) you.

Staying Open-Minded

I would also like to point out here how a small thing can make a big difference. When I was on the gluten-free diet, I was told in order for a product to be gluten free it had to have less than twenty parts per million.[12] Per million! I was incredibly diligent about avoiding cross-contamination because of this. So, we played this *food game* very close to our chest. We never ate out. I made the entire family go gluten free. It was just easier and safer.

I remember when I started researching a gluten-free, casein-free diet for my autistic son. Living in a small town in the middle of nowhere, Montana, bookstores were where we went for entertainment. The only book I could find was *Living Gluten Free for Dummies* by Danna Korn. As I read it, I saw my mom on those pages. I saw me on those pages. I felt like I was reading the medical records of my family. I confess, the author irritated me a little. (It seemed like she implied it was because we went overboard on breads and pastas. For me, I was told by my doctor during my first pregnancy that I needed to eat more of it. Yuck!) I wondered how this small factor of gluten could be possible.

They said the two ways to tell would be to either have a test done or to go without for a period of time. I chose the latter. On day five, I was shocked. People can feel this good? I never knew. I was curious. I avoided gluten for the whole

---

[12] Food and Drug Administration. "Gluten and Food Labeling." FDA. Content current as of 16 July 2018. https://www.fda.gov/food/nutrition-education-resources-materials/gluten-and-food-labeling.

family, all eight of us, for two weeks. My toddler, who never spoke, started talking in full sentences. ALL OF THE TIME! His personality was hidden under gluten. Again, can I say shocked!? Two of my kids grew over six inches each in the following months. My autistic son started coming out of the clouds. He was giving us sustained eye contact.

I was sold. I was also mad. The doctors knew my son was autistic. Why did they never tell me? Heck, they knew I cooked with whole grain wheat and made our tortillas and bread from scratch—trying to do the Feingold diet (no food additives or preservatives) the best we could.

Fast-forward, we were on the GF diet. Some of us egg and dairy free, as well. Others, soy free or corn free. For three solid years, not a single cheat. People would say it must be hard. Yes and no. Yes, it was hard preparing meals for so many different needs. And no. For how much it affected our health, nothing could taste good enough to make it worth the cheat.

Fast-forward again, we no longer follow any strict diets. We don't need to. In fact, when I was trying to explain this to a doctor of mine, she was convinced gluten was the problem. I told her it was no longer an issue. She said those types of allergies never really go away. She wasn't going to help me until I went back on the diet. I agreed to an allergy test. I even made sure I ate both gluten and dairy before taking the test. The allergy test confirmed dairy and gluten were a nonissue. Now it was her turn to be shocked and confused. I also loved her honesty. She said she didn't know how to help me then, but she would love to help me in any way she could.

Going Forward Alone

I heard this wonderful word of advice the other day. It was meant for a photographer. A photographer who was stuck. He felt like his pictures looked like everybody else's pictures. He wanted his work to stick out. The advice given to him was to just stay on the train longer than everyone else and he would see things nobody else has seen. All the photographers were getting on at point A and getting off at point B. He decided to stay on the train when everyone else got off. His photography business exploded!

I guess you could say I stayed on the train, mainly because I wasn't allowed to get off.

➢ I went to my OB/GYN. He couldn't help me. So, I was on my own.

➢ I started looking for answers myself through books. It led me to the GFCF egg-free diet. I hit a wall. I needed help over this new wall.

➢ I went to a naturopathic doctor. She found the pituitary gland problem. She helped me over that wall. She helped me until she couldn't anymore. What was supposed to be working wasn't. Treating my pituitary gland was causing me to be weaker and develop many more food allergies. The wall had become too tall. She suggested acupuncture and homeopathy.

➢ I went to an acupuncturist, homeopath, and chiropractor until that no longer worked. Meanwhile, still on what would be called an MS (multiple sclerosis) Diet Plan. No gluten, eggs, soy, casein, preservatives, corn, etc.

➢ My acupuncturist said she was at the end of her knowledge. Big wall. Do I sit down? No, instead she pushed me up. She shared her knowledge with me. I asked her so many questions, for three years. I used her information and flipped it totally upside down. I climbed over this new wall and continued down the path alone.

➢ This is when I decided to start back at the very beginning and assume the only thing I knew to be true. Like waves canceled. But they have to be an exact match. I was sure of nothing else.

➢ I started to improve.

I am now sure I figured out something we aren't aware of. This something explained why what was supposed to work wasn't working for me.

Topic 2: What We Are and Aren't Told

The Common Ground

There are many approaches and views about how to treat an illness. There are also numerous views of what constitutes a healthy lifestyle. Regardless of your location on this medical spectrum, I think we can safely agree most are advocates for a healthful lifestyle. I think we can also safely agree the whole body is involved in a person's health, both physically and mentally. With those two basic principles in mind, we have the agreed big picture of what I'll call the Big Five Assumptions for Health.

The Big Five Assumptions for Health

1. Diet: A restricted diet (pick one) of some sort. Many people would swear by the one they are on. BUT, it doesn't work for everyone. In fact, the healthier I ate, the more food allergies I developed!

The mathematician in me thought 2 + 2 is true because it is always 4. If proper diet was the key, why doesn't it work for everyone?

2. Exercise: I made every effort I could to keep my body moving. If pregnant, I was walking all the time. If not pregnant, biking, hiking, skating, martial arts, stretching, or swimming. Just do something every day.

3. Reduce Stress: I did not have a stressful life. I loved my life. I even started using Dr. Bradley Nelson's *The Emotion*

Code[13] protocol just in case emotions had anything to do with it and I just wasn't aware of it.

4. Avoid Bad Guys: As you recall, Bad Guys is going to be my terminology for the pathogens, viruses, bacteria, chemicals, you name it, whatever causes harm to the body. The culprits who shouldn't be there. I did everything I could here, but I couldn't control what happened to me in my childhood or before I was born.

5. Avoid Inflammation: Some do this with medication. I understand taking anti-inflammatory drugs is a common practice. A necessary evil even. Been there, done that. But shouldn't it be a red flag to us? Suppressing an immune system when the immune system is what fixes the body. I know, for some, it just has to be done. It is a no-win scenario. Others may avoid inflammation with diet or supplements. They blame having the wrong diet for the inflammation.

What if... we have this backwards? Or a little tipped.

Are We Assuming Wrong?

For example, exercising. When they did research, they noticed healthy people exercised regularly. Researchers concluded exercising needed to be a part of a healthy person's life.[14]

---

[13] Nelson, Dr. Bradley. *The Emotion Code* (Wellness Unmasked Publishing, 2007).

[14] Harvard Health Publishing: Harvard Medical School. "The Secret to Better Health—Exercise." Harvard College. 6 March 2012. https://www.health.harvard.edu/healthbeat/the-secret-to-better-health-exercise.

Thus, the conclusion: in order to be healthy, one needed to exercise regularly. But isn't this an assumption? All they really knew was that healthy people exercised, and unhealthy people didn't.

- We are told to exercise.
  - Some exercise but still fall victim to health challenges. Why?
  - Some are advised not to exercise—what can they do then?
- If most people know they should exercise, why don't they?

My personal experience has been that when I felt good, it was difficult to get me to not exercise. And when I wasn't feeling good, it took incredible willpower to put in the work anyway. And this idea of exercising seems to be taking a shift now. The parameters seem to be changing on what constitutes *enough* productive exercising.

Another example is stress. I think we are making an assumption here as well. We are concluding it is stress. Stress causes high cortisol levels, so if I have high cortisol levels, I must be stressed.

What if... something else was causing the high cortisol levels?

What if... these high cortisol levels made it easier to become stressed? Or maybe being stressed wasn't the problem but being unable to reduce the cortisol levels was.

What if... something was preventing the cortisol levels from being able to normalize?

What if... something was preventing the cortisol from being able to be removed from my body?

I know I'm running the risk of sounding like a broken record here, but if I was doing those five things and my health still prevented me from functioning normally on a daily basis, what else is there left to do? Do those five things AND... what?

What is missing?

If I say genetics, then do I just throw in the towel? My will to live wouldn't let me.

A Word on Pain

Pain is my body's way of telling me something is wrong. Fix it. But we have come to conclude that it means to take something so I don't feel it. I think we have started doing this with inflammation as well. The body is trying to tell us something is wrong. We focus on the pain or the inflammation. We focus on removing the symptoms. We see the symptoms as the problem, so we make the symptoms go away. However, the problem is still there.

Why did the problem show up in the first place?

Because of an X.

But why?

Because it does Y to the body.

But why?

Yes, I was the annoying person who asked all the questions. In fact, when giving out nicknames in Officer Training School, I was given the nickname "Mrs. I Have a Question." (True story.)

Another example. In acupuncture, I was told pain meant blockage. My question was, "But what is causing the blockage?" Good question to ask. But what if this was backwards? Maybe, sometimes, well at least for me, I found I needed to take it a step further back. I needed to look at it like pain and inflammation. I needed to determine if the blockage was the problem or if what was *causing* the blockage was. What if the body was trying to protect itself from something worse and therefore causing the blockage for my protection? What do I mean by something worse? What if, when the body was fighting to remove the harmful problem, it was taking with it something the body needed?

Our Organs

If we think about doing a workout, who sweats the most? (Assuming you are not one of those people who doesn't sweat.) Two types of people do. One is the person who is very out of shape doing a light workout. The other person is in really good shape trying to do an intense workout. When we become ill, I think we tend to believe it is because of the first scenario. Our organs are just ka-pluey and we need to whip them into shape. Maybe that isn't always the case. Maybe it is the other guy. Maybe as a person's body becomes stronger, it decides to try to lift the heavy barbell over its proverbial head because it thought it could do it now. But just because it thought it could, doesn't mean it could. Maybe this is what goes wrong.

I just know, for me, it got ugly before it got better. And it got really ugly when I was at the height of my healthful lifestyle. Why? Wouldn't it make sense that the more rules I followed, the healthier I would be?

Disagreements

Since we can't all agree on the solution, I would like to propose "the field" to connect many of the paths together. We know inflammation causes problems with many diseases. We also know high cortisol levels contribute to health challenges as well. Instead of focusing on the illnesses these two factors cause, what if we focus on the possibility of removing them from the equation?

What I want to share with you in this book worked for me over and over again. It explains a different approach to the inflammation problem. It also helped me to reduce my cortisol levels immediately. It eliminated pain. It is a simple concept, but it is not easy. Sometimes it is a quick fix, but since I was learning as I was going, it was sometimes hard to find the missing piece to the puzzle. But once it was found, the results were felt within hours. This puzzle piece required me to do something with it over a period of time ranging from four days to fifteen months.

Topic 3: What We Have Noticed or Experienced

Health, religion, and politics all have one thing in common: people have their convictions and their extreme views on how it should be done. Sometimes it is easy to miss the point of both views having the same objective. Instead of focusing on *what should be done*, let's focus on the end goal. For well-being, it would be improved health for everybody. But something is wrong. What we know about health doesn't work for everyone. Why is that?

Information

1. **Conflicting Information**

I think this might be why it is so difficult sometimes to do what is considered beneficial to our health. We are warned about environmental hazards. It would logically make sense to tell my doctor about them when exposure did happen. My experience, for the most part, has been that when I have brought my exposure concerns up to my doctor, they were dismissed. Why? Should it be a concern or not?

2. **Withheld Information**

Why did my doctor, who knew my son was on the autism spectrum, fail to tell us about the gluten-free diet? She knew we wanted to know how to help him naturally. Why did we have to stumble on this information ourselves? When we mentioned it to her at our next doctor visit, she knew about it! What?! FYI: eliminating egg eliminated the violent tantrums. Eliminating dairy caused him to go through almost druglike addiction withdrawals for four days. Eliminating gluten stimulated quicker hair growth and added inches to his frame at a rapid rate.

3. Limited Information

In antibody testing, it can only tell us what the body has fought. It can't tell if it is still fighting. For me, testing for lymphatic parasites would have been pointless. I had tested positive in the past. It can't tell me if I'm still fighting them. Or worse, what if the Bad Guy is there but the body is unable to fight it? This, too, would not show up on the test.

An entire book could be written on this next sentence, but I want to stay on point. Tests may not be reliable.[15] Said, done. Moving on. False positive and false negative results are equally bad. If the symptoms my doctor was seeing weren't lining up with the test results, we were both stuck. If you're a doctor, you could be in a bunch of trouble if you still proceed against what the test results said. Should the doctors trust their eyes or the results more?

Pseudoscience Accusations

There will always be naysayers. But instead of jumping on this boat so quickly, maybe we should visit the idea that science just hasn't caught up yet to what we are noticing. Sometimes we see results. Sometimes we don't. Is what I am going to share in this book a contributing factor to why this is the case? It was for me. So, please, instead of practitioners assuming we aren't doing the work of the Big Five, or that we fail to believe the suggested methods work, hear me out to the end of my argument.

---

[15] Cecchini, Cherilyn, MD. "How Accurate Are Your Lab Results? Here's What You Need to Know." GoodRx Health. Updated on 8 February 2023. https://www.goodrx.com/health-topic/diagnostics/how-accurate-are-my-lab-test-results.

1. Homeopathy & Herbs

These forms of medicine have not only been around longer than modern medicine, but modern medicine has used them to try to build off them. For example, salicylic acid, from the willow tree, is how they discovered a way to make aspirin.[16] Creating it artificially was the only way to keep up with the demand for it. If someone tells you aspirin is safe because it is natural, they are wrong. It may be safe, but it is not natural (derived from the willow tree). I personally feel like it is the same as saying instant and old-school mashed potatoes are the same. They are not.

There are more examples than this. Aspirin just happens to be the most widely known one. Yams were studied for birth control,[17] and essential oils are currently being studied for antibiotic-resistant infections.[18] I've even heard about bloodletting still taking place. Why are they revisiting and/or using these unless there is something to it?[19]

---

[16] LeCouteur, Penny, and Jay Burreson. *Napoleon's Buttons* (Jeremy P. Tarcher/Penguin, 2003), 183.

[17] LeCouteur, Burreson. *Napoleon's Buttons*, 211.

[18] Yap, Polly Soo Xi, Swee Hua Erin Lim, Cai Ping Hu, and Beow Chin Yiap. "Combination of Essential Oils and Antibiotics Reduce Antibiotic Resistance in Plasmid-Conferred Multidrug Resistant Bacteria." National Library of Medicine. 26 March 2013. https://pubmed.ncbi.nlm.nih.gov/23537749/.

[19] Nierenberg, Cari. "10 'Barbaric' Medical Treatments That Are Still Used Today." Live Science. 5 August 2016.

2. Sway Testing

Sway testing is a skill. It can be learned. It is not all inclusive, but neither are many medical tests. But the more I practiced this skill, the better at it I became. Practitioners with over five years of experience have an accuracy rate of ninety-eight percent.[20] I say impressive. Sway testing was the only tool I had at my disposal. If I had a more sophisticated machine available, maybe I would have used it. I don't know. But having the ability and skill to sway test did allow me to take control of my health. Sway testing helped because it allowed me to make the smallest of adjustments in my environment and diet to enable me to improve. Best of all, it was immediate. No waiting weeks to see what to do next. A lot can happen in those weeks to where the results may no longer even be accurate. I know, not one hundred percent accurate, but what test is?

> A side note here for those who think it is quite odd for the body to know what it does and does not need.
>
> Study microbiology.
>
> The body knows...

3. Acupuncture

If you aren't familiar with acupuncture, it is the process of using a variety of needles in a variety of angles and methods

---

https://www.livescience.com/55667-barbaric-medical-treatments-still-used.html.

[20] Abrams, Joel. "Muscle Testing (Kinesiology): Panacea or Placebo?" The Conversation. 18 December 2012. https://theconversation.com/muscle-testing-kinesiology-panacea-or-placebo-11075.

to target what is called acupuncture points in the body to aid or correct energy flow so a person can heal and recover properly on their own. Let's just say this technique has been used for centuries. With that being said, even so, they didn't prove meridians and acupuncture points existed until 2016.[21] They have called it the primo-vascular system. Talk about a lag in science catching up...

Willing to Try Anything

Many a countless time when my physical ability to function like everyone else could not be caroused on a given day, the tendency was to dismiss it as a change in the weather, that time of the month, just being upset, stressed, overdoing it, imagining it, or exaggerating my symptoms. You name it. I'm sure you have heard them all. I'm also sure, if you are like me, you started doubting yourself and questioning whether to believe them all. Maybe even thinking, *It's just me. What is my problem?*

But alas, those repeated dismissals eventually add up and suddenly a decade or two of life has gone by. I was finally told what was wrong. (Most chronic illnesses take years to be diagnosed.[22]) It's not because I kept looking until I had

---

[21] Martin, Charles. "Auburn Scientist Discovers Microstructure of Primo-Vascular System, Revealing Possible Foundation of How Acupuncture Works." Auburn University. 1 December 2016. https://ocm.auburn.edu/newsroom/news_articles/2016/12/auburn-scientist-discovers-microstructure-of-primo-vascular-system.php.

[22] Benness, Brianne. "The 5 Stages of a Chronic-Illness Diagnosis." Elemental. 12 November 2019. https://elemental.medium.com/diagnosis-is-a-process-not-an-event-db1e6ae2ac35.

something wrong. It was because the one who continued to look for the needle in the haystack was the one whose life was being slowly sucked away with no help in sight. I knew something was there because I was being continually reminded of it when I needed to lie down and rest after only taking a shower.

Einstein said, "Everything should be made as simple as possible, but not simpler."

When I did finally figure out what I plan to share with you in this book, I was shocked at how simple the concept was. I wondered how often this could be the case for others as well. I looked at other health problems. I would notice many times when the idea was carried out to this new conclusion, it made sense. It was connected. Fascinating. If I looked at the problems through these new glasses, the connections were very visible. It made me start wondering if we were seeing our health problems backwards.

Well, this new concept I discovered was easy. However, the implementation of it was very difficult to learn. In the end, I was able to tie up all the loose ends to where it made logical sense to me. I am not a doctor or a professional scientist. I don't have a group of peers to give me a peer review or publish my findings. Heck, some of you might even think I have no right to write this book. But write it, I will. I must. I think this is valuable information.

Let's just say I am more of a medical philosopher. I am asking you to think differently. To think backwards for a little while. Back when Copernicus and the scientists of ancient days were around, they would publish what they observed to the general public. They would let the people decide for themselves what to think. Well, that is what I am doing here. I am inviting you to think for yourself instead of having someone tell you what you need to think.

What if chronic inflammation is

just the check engine light?

I am not the historian who knows about all the different key battles, maneuvers, spies, and motives behind the war. I am the lowly soldier in the trenches who saw it firsthand. I know what I saw, and I know what I experienced. My goal is not to contradict but to illuminate. To be the key decoder. To show how it is all connected. We already knew it was, but here is another piece to close the gaps even more. If what I know is truly what is happening, prevention alone could take us far.

Personal Examples

What I Tried

At one point, I had read SO MANY books on how the body worked and what I needed to do for my body to function properly. I was exhausted. If those were true, it would have worked by now for sure. But it hadn't. I was so tired of trying. So tired of getting my hopes up and thinking, *Oh, that is what I didn't consider. That is what the problem was*. But, alas, no. Meanwhile, I was continually seeking help from all the methods previously mentioned.

We are told to leave it to the experts, but if they don't know the answers, is it wrong to try to find them ourselves? I don't think so. So that is what I did.

Sometimes, it is very difficult not to get really angry when I think back on it. The bridge was out ahead, and I knew it was. I kept trying to warn everyone and they wouldn't listen. The bridge ends up going out and they say, "Look, your problem is that the bridge is out." Ugh!

Because of this, I guess you could say I had placed myself into a category called "Not-Me." It seemed, even though it worked for others, it didn't work for me. It seemed like it didn't matter what it was. In case you were wondering what I had already tried, I've included my list. When I mean tried, I mean a minimum of six months' effort for each method, usually years, and in many combinations. It was so complicated. How should I know what to do? What to try? How long to try it for? When to give up? Should I give up? Should I accept my verdict? Should I just quit trying and say I gave it a *good 'ole college effort*? If it were just me, I probably would have. But, looking at my two-year-old, I knew God would provide her with a new mom or mother-figure if it was to be, but I wanted it to be me. So, I kept trying.

It Doesn't Work for Everyone

In spite of all these efforts, the hard truth is it doesn't work for everyone. When it doesn't, mistrust develops between doctor and patient. The doctor thinks the patient isn't being totally honest and the patient doesn't think the doctor is listening or believing them. Sometimes the patient is accused of being too sensitive or making a bigger deal out of her health problems than other people do. Or worst of all, she is believed to be making it up. Hello, maybe she is just trying to zero in on what is wrong so she can live her life to the fullest again.

<u>It Wasn't From Lack of Trying...</u>

- Probiotics
- Enzymes
- Parasite Cleanse
- Master Cleanse
- Candida Diet
- Essential Oils
- Massage
- Exams
- Tests
- Medication
- Shots
- Exercise
- Chiropractor
- Acupuncture
- NAET
- Supplements
- GFCF egg-free Diet
- Raw Diet (very difficult by the way when allergic to sunflower seeds and bananas)
- Other Diets
- Stress Reduction
- Emotion Code
- Magnets
- Miracle Mineral Solution
- Homeopathy
- Adequate Water Consumption
- Prayer

And the list goes on...

Pause here: Someone invented a menstrual belt and a labor belt to enable men to feel what it is like to endure what is common routine for women. Wouldn't it be nice if they could invent something similar to this for chronic pain or fatigue sufferers? Maybe we are the tough ones after all.

Thought to Ponder

- If diet and exercise was the fix, wouldn't some form of diet and exercise routine fix everyone?
- We seem to learn more and more about diets and our bodies. Why isn't this knowledge being reflected in the health status of the nation?
- Do you know someone who doesn't even know the definition of the word *healthy?* Yes, an exaggeration, yet they are.
- Do you know someone who is obsessed with diet and exercise and yet they still fell prey to disease?
- Yes, I know everyone dies, but do you understand my point? Why are these the case?
- Is there something else going on we aren't aware of?
- Is there a way to recover and survive in our chemical-laden world?
- Do you or someone you know have an example of an event in their life that changed their health?
- We are told the value of a healthy gut and the dangers of pathogens. What if healthfulness was not on this sliding scale but an entire other piece was missing to tie it all together?
- Are you slowly giving up more of your life and joys so you can function and make it through the day?

- Are you walking around with an invisible illness because something invisible is stealing your well-being away?

Conclusion for Chapter 2

I have not blown off all we have learned about germs, diseases, and the human body. I am familiar with it all. However, when the Big Five Assumptions weren't working for me, I knew I needed to get a different perspective. I needed to look at good health from a different angle. The only way I could do that was to go as far back as I could to see if I could find a different trailhead that may have been hidden before. I needed to build off what we already knew but with as few assumptions as possible. For example...

Autoimmune Diseases

More than 23.5 million Americans have an autoimmune disease.[23] I have heard some people argue the tests are just more accurate now. However, even scientists will admit that, though this is possible, it is highly unlikely[24] because there is

---

[23] U.S. Department of Health and Human Services, Office on Women's Health. "Autoimmune Diseases." U.S. Department of Health and Human Services. Last updated 22 February 2021. https://www.womenshealth.gov/a-z-topics/autoimmune-diseases.

[24] Love, Tessa. "Why Are Autoimmune Diseases on the Rise?" Elemental. 10 April 2019. https://elemental.medium.com/autoimmunity-is-a-disorder-of-our-time-a7f1c45d6907#:~:text=It%E2%80%99s%20possible%20that%20the%20apparent%20increase%20in%20autoimmune,of%20autoimmunity.%20Something%20else%20must%20be%20at%20play.

even an increase in the diseases that have been very easy to diagnose in the past, such as type 1 diabetes.[25]

Here is a list of the common traits for autoimmune diseases:

- Industrialized countries
- Genetics
- Environment
- Infectious agents
- Hormones
- Viruses (especially Epstein Barr)
- "Something" happened, and the body is now attacking itself.

Is it possible this *something that happened* could be as simple as hormones becoming combined with an environmental toxin or virus to where the body can no longer fight to remove the Bad Guy because it is taking the Good Guy with it causing inflammation? Is it possible? Yes. Is it probable? I don't know. But let's at least look in that direction for an answer.

Looking at the assumption of "something happened, and the body is now attacking itself" seemed like a good starting point. I saw it happen to me. But I got to thinking about how problems are usually the outward manifestation of something that happened earlier. The real question should be what was different between the before and after of "something happening."

[25] Polonsky, Kenneth S., MD. "The Past 200 Years in Diabetes." *New England Journal of Medicine*. 4 October 2012. https://www.nejm.org/doi/full/10.1056/NEJMra1110560.

CHAPTER 3:

A DIFFERENT VANTAGE POINT

It is possible we have it backwards.

Opening Story: Trying to Correct My Pituitary Gland

As I mentioned, my whole family went gluten free. My autistic son and I went GFCF egg free. His health improved. My health improved for the first three months. It then started declining. More food allergies, more fatigue, more downcast feelings, more confusion about why it was not working for me. I went to a naturopath to try and figure out a way to fix the years of damage gluten may have caused me. She had me taking many very high doses of different supplements. It didn't help.

She ran a test, we waited for the results—nothing. Ran another test, waited for the results—still nothing. She said I was low on testosterone and she gave me something for it. I didn't buy it. I asked her, "And if it isn't this, if this doesn't work, then what?" She said she would test my pituitary gland. I said, "Test me." She wanted to wait and see if the medication she suggested would work first. I said, "No, test me. I'll start the medication, but test me." She reluctantly did and was shocked by the results. We immediately started four shots a week on the actual human growth hormone, not the one that stimulates it.

Did I get better? No. My health plummeted even further. I gained new food allergies daily. My winter coat and boots were too heavy to wear, so I quit going outside. My head felt like it was on fire. I couldn't sleep anymore. I went from *Tae Kwon Do* workouts to not being able to walk around the block. These shots were destroying my life, but my numbers were too low. I really had no choice but to do them.

Looking back now, it is clear to me. We had this backwards to a degree. My low human growth hormone was not the problem. My problem was causing low human growth hormone levels. Forcing these levels up when the body was trying to protect me by keeping them down triggered all the other problems to the point of me being recommended to test for multiple sclerosis.

Overview

I think a major problem we have is we can't seem to agree on the correct solution. We have a wide spectrum of one extreme of medicine (modern medicine) to the other extreme of what doesn't seem to look like medicine at all (alternative medicine). Somewhere in the middle lies integrative medicine. I would think somewhere on this sliding scale results could be found. But, alas, people still fall through the cracks. I fell through the cracks.

I am going to make a bold statement here and say, if the real solution was found, wouldn't it work for everyone somehow on this sliding scale? Wouldn't it be easier to believe in the validity of the claims if they were consistent? But they aren't, are they? This drug, diet, procedure, treatment works for X, but then the disclaimers come for all the possible side effects and inconsistent results for the Y and Z people. And ever notice, the Y and Z people seem to always be the same type of people? They always seem to be the ones who need it the most but are unable to do it. Maybe. Or maybe I am just being biased here because the one it didn't work for was always me.

Because of this category of people who either had X not work or didn't want to take the risk of the side effects to try, like me, they decide to go someplace else to play. To look for different answers to their questions. This might be why a number of people turn to alternative means even if they hadn't been raised in the culture. The other ways weren't working or may have been too risky. But even the box of alternatives is so overwhelming. So many options. Where to start? What to do? How long do I continue to try before I try something else? Results vary, of course. How to know if I'm varying within the parameters of progress forward?

- What if... there was only one missing piece?
- What if... figuring out this so-called health matrix enabled any method to work?
- What if... this matrix could truly merge the philosophies by seeing how they worked together?
- What if... this missing piece has been in plain sight the whole time and we just never made the connection of what the ramifications of it were?
- What if... understanding this one malfunction of the body contributed to correcting SO many problems?

If this malfunction is the cause of inflammation and inflammation is the cause of so many problems with diseases, fixing the one malfunction, however I choose, should fix the problem.

Do we dare hope?

Do we dare look?

Do we dare make the viruses of the world powerless against us?

Colin Powell was quoted as saying, "If everyone is thinking alike, then somebody isn't thinking."

Well, here is my challenge to you to think outside of the box. I do not claim I have it all figured out. In fact, I'll freely admit, I'm still learning. I just can't wait any longer to share what I do know so far. I chose to be my own guinea pig and start with the only truth I knew had no contradictions to it. Like waves canceled. (If you want to research it, it is called destructive interference.) I slowly progressed from there.

- What if... we had a body system we already knew about, which was doing something we didn't know it was doing?
- What if... the difference between being someone who can have success with a treatment and someone who cannot is this system going awry?
- What if... there was a way to manually override and reprogram this system until the body was able to do it without additional assistance anymore?

Topic 1: Taking a Step Back

Back to the example in the book *Blink* of the one who knows less being able to see it more clearly. I don't know the stacks of medical book knowledge of what is going on. I am not the expert in this labyrinth of knowledge going deep into the recesses of so many places about the human body. But because of this lack of knowledge, maybe it was easier for me to see the big picture. I didn't get bogged down with all the details. Maybe my not knowing where to look caused me to look in different and unexpected places. The experiences my body was having were making my brain scream for understanding of what was happening. Why couldn't I be like everyone else and find something that worked for me?

Circling the Problem

What came first, the chicken or the egg? Some say chicken, some say egg, but everybody can agree there is a chicken AND an egg. The only way anyone can definitively say one or the other came first is by making assumptions. This applies in so many areas of illnesses. I would like to just focus on gluten as an example.

I was affected by gluten. When I cut it out of my diet, it made such a difference, I actually struggled with anger for some time for not having been told about it sooner. But me and my questions got me going again. Why? The answers I would get made sense. But I still kept adding, *but why?*

Issues with gluten caused health problems. Okay... but what if the health problems caused the gluten challenges? It could happen. Logically, if celiac-gluten intolerance can come on anytime, then something happened to make it come on.

So, can something happen to also make it go away? More questions.

According to Liverdoctor.com, "It is estimated that eighty percent of alcoholics are gluten intolerant. Alcoholics improve greatly when all grains and gluten products are removed from their diets."[26] They speculate that the gluten sensitivity may be more the cause of addiction than the alcohol itself. Others on the internet are looking into alcohol dependency as being the cause of gluten issues.[27] Questions, questions, questions.

I think we can all see there is a strong possibility of them being connected to each other. But instead of playing the game of which came first, let's ask why they are connected in the first place.

Knowing the Problem

It is impossible to live in the world today without hearing about germ theory and viruses. There are over 200 different types of viruses that can infect humans.[28] Some of these

---

[26] Liver Doctor. "Alcoholism—Hypoglycaemia—Gluten Intolerance." Liver Doctor. Last accessed 27 March 2023. https://www.liverdoctor.com/alcoholism-hypoglycaemia-gluten-intolerance/.

[27] Hess, Christopher P., ed. "Alcohol Induces Sensitization to Gluten in Genetically Susceptible Individuals: A Case Control Study." National Library of Medicine. 15 October 2013. https://www.ncbi.nlm.nih.gov/pmc/articles/PMC3817350/.

[28] WebMD. "What's Causing My Cold?" WebMD. Reviewed 5 May 2021. https://www.webmd.com/cold-and-flu/cold-guide/common_cold_causes.

viruses can even cause cancer.[29] Even so, two people can be exposed to the same virus, and one person can die from it while the other person is either asymptomatic or fails to become infected at all. What gives?

Maybe it is because we also need to include the condition of our guts. There are many things that can be done to help us with this. There are already many books out there about it. But... getting my body to acknowledge my efforts was a different story. I ate probiotics like candy and was on an eighty percent raw diet with the rest being a candida limiting diet. No luck.

I had a virus(es) in me and a gut that wouldn't help me in spite of all the assisting I could do for it. Was there one more thing I could do? I was willing. Maybe there was a threesome here we just hadn't considered yet. Maybe.

My Suggestion

I would like to propose that maybe there are two categories of people. Maybe these two categories of people need to be treated differently. What if dealing with these two categories differently enabled already existing procedures, medicines, supplements, and treatments to actually do their job for this

---

[29] American Cancer Society medical and editorial content team. "Viruses That Can Lead to Cancer." American Cancer Society. Last revised 21 March 2023. https://www.cancer.org/healthy/cancer-causes/infectious-agents/infections-that-can-lead-to-cancer/viruses.html.

alienated group? You know, the group addressed with the *really fast words* at the end of all those drug commercials? Doesn't it always seem to be the ones who need the help the most that are the ones unable to *be* helped?

Fishbowl Analogy

Let's say we have two round fishbowls—the kind you see in cartoons all the time. We placed a quart of water in both. However, one had a crack preventing the bowl from ever being able to hold more than half a quart of water. We put one fish in each bowl. Let's say an outside circumstance happened that neither one had any control over. Let's say it caused the first fishbowl to lose half of its water. It also caused the cracked bowl to lose the same amount of water. I think we could safely suspect the fish in the originally full bowl didn't really care about what happened. Nothing seemed different. He was not hindered at all in his trips back and forth in his bowl from one side to the other. I also suspect the second fish in the cracked bowl probably became a little bit stressed about the situation.

If you use your imagination, you could probably see the first fish swimming around asking the other fish what he is so stressed about. Big deal, so half of our water was dumped. No need to get upset. Meanwhile the second fish wants to believe him but is having trouble swimming in the bowl because his top fin is sticking out of the water and his tummy is rubbing on the rocks. "Okay, you're right, I'm making a big deal out of nothing. I'll continue to go about my business in spite of my difficulties because everyone is telling me it is what I need to do." Maybe he damages a fin, scratches off a few scales, or has trouble getting around. Maybe he is even short of breath. So, both tanks get filled up again to where they were before. The second fish will think, *Everything is as it was before; I must be making a big deal out of nothing*. He again swims around as he originally did. Damaged perhaps, but he will mend. He is oblivious to the fact that his water loss was a bit different than the first fish experiencing the same thing. He believes the first fish is right. He thinks he needs to toughen up.

The first fish is equated with those who are on path A. They are able to do the recommended protocol to improve their health. The second fish is on path B. He did not choose to start with a half empty bowl. In fact, he wasn't even aware of it. It was all he has ever known. He thinks what he experiences is the same as fish A. He just needed to deal with things differently, like the first fish did. But he can't. He thinks he must be handling something wrong to be so upset about having his bowl emptied. The other fish didn't seem to mind. Why should he? Maybe everyone else is right. Maybe? No! And yes.

Depending on the different fields of medicine, fish B may be classified as someone with a weak immune system, a poor constitution, or a weak or "blocked" energy field. They are blaming the fish for the problem. They think something is wrong with the fish. What I am here to suggest is that maybe there is an entire system in our body causing some people to have a cracked bowl. The cracked bowl goes unnoticed because we never realized it was even there. The cracked bowl is the problem, not the fish.

Getting Clarity

What do I know? By taking a step back, I noticed doing these *five healthful things* didn't work. I was still missing something. Was it because I had no choice in the matter? This is what I got stuck with so this is what I have to be like. Unacceptable. My logical brain was quite sure we were missing something. Time to search again with a finer-toothed comb, so to speak. Let's revisit the Big Five Health Assumptions without including the chicken vs. the egg scenario.

Reworded to be the Big Five Health *Challenges*

1. **Why Diet:** Nutrition matters.
2. **Why Exercise:** A healthy body is a moving body.
3. **Why Stress:** Need lower cortisol levels.
4. **Why Avoid Bad Guys:** Easier on the organs.
5. **Why Avoid Inflammation:** Don't want body to attack itself.

I started with what I did know. I knew nutrition mattered. Period. I wasn't going to assume anything else past that. I do know that in spite of all my efforts, my body was not getting or using these nutrients. And yes, I did go down all those traditional rabbit holes searching for the causes of this. Came up empty handed. I almost gave up on it all when, after consuming large quantities of probiotics over a year and a half while doing the candida diet protocol, the flora in my gut did not change AT ALL. At all!? I figured this probably had quite a bit to do with all the other health challenges. But knowing it needed fixing and fixing it were two totally different situations. If I continued to focus on it, it wouldn't work. It wasn't going to fix anything because it hadn't caused any change yet. I needed to focus somewhere else.

The Day When Everything Changed

After aggressively pursuing alternative medicine options for over four years, I eventually came to a time where I said I give up. I didn't know what else to do. I call it Hell Week now looking back. To me, an excellent definition of hell is ***no hope***. The night before Hell Week began, I felt better than I had in years. I had such clarity of thought. My pen couldn't go fast enough to get all my thoughts on paper while I was sitting in the sauna that Sunday evening. When I returned home, I spent a terrific evening with the family. I thought, yes, this is going to work this time.

The very next morning it began—so dizzy, so nauseous. The only way to get relief from it was to either be soaking in the tub with remedies or biking for hours at a time on my stationary bike. If I wasn't doing one or the other, I felt like I was going to pass out. By Friday I was exhausted. But this was not the low point. I lost control of my right leg. It was like it had a mind of its own. It was moving all over the place like a cat trying to get the tape off the bottom of its paw. It was like it couldn't receive the signals my body wanted it to receive.

I went to the acupuncturist I had been going to regularly for the past three years. She put one needle into the bottom of my foot, which was still trying to not be held still. With that contact, my soul began to wail with such deep and loud crying I had never experienced before. I had no idea where it was coming from. When it was over, I was in a pool of sweat. She said it was an emotional release. Fine, but it didn't fix anything. The dizziness was still there. The leg shaking was still there. And I would later learn, the screaming was still there. The screaming was so loud, and I couldn't stop it. I felt like if I did, I would die. It was like what they refer to in *Tae Kwon Do* as a *kihap*, a spirit cry. It scared me. I know it scared my kids too. But even my maternal instincts to protect them couldn't stop the hysteria bolting from my body.

After this happened again a third time, I allowed my husband to take me to the emergency room. They couldn't find (surprise, surprise, not) what was wrong. I had to stay the night to make sure. When I came home the following day, I ended up complying with my husband's request. He told me to stop taking the homeopathic remedies. Stop taking—stop doing the *only thing* that seemed to help at all? I was devastated and felt like he'd just slammed the hammer down on my death sentence. I could understand why he said what he said, but it still cut like a knife. Oddly enough, this "mean act" enabled me to figure out what I needed to do. I don't think I would have figured this out if he hadn't done that. Sometimes God works in mysterious ways. (Getting ahead of myself. It's coming up.)

Topic 2: Starting Over

Being Cut Off

So, with Hell Week under my belt, I felt utterly alone. I was cut off from my homeopath and acupuncturist. I succumbed to taking the doctor-prescribed medicines. In return, it fixed nothing. It only became worse. I was allowed to add insomnia, sleep apnea, and abdominal pain to my problems. Worst of all, I had lost hope of anybody listening to me. I cried and didn't sleep for a month—the severe sleep apnea the new medicine brought on made sure of that. The medicines fixed nothing. Now what? Give up or go it alone? I'd been a lone wolf before; I guessed this was no different. I separated from the pack.

I was not only all the way back to square one again. I was worse. However, this time I did have more knowledge. Somewhere in the pit of my stomach, I knew the answer was in front of me. I just couldn't see it yet. Right then and there, I made a decision, a resolve. I was going to clear my name. My emotional state was not causing my illness. They had it backwards. My illness was causing my emotional state.

I started over, but differently. I broke it down into even smaller pieces. I looked even deeper and in different places. I assumed as little as possible. I had to think outside the box in order to get out of the box I was placed in.

Finding Solid Ground

I went back to the very beginning. I started with the most simple and obvious things to me. I came up with four.

1. I knew muscle testing (sway testing) worked. Maybe it wasn't a perfect science, but the more I used it, the more accurate it became.

2. I knew meridians in the body affected my health.

3. I knew homeopathic remedies affected those meridians.

[Homeopathy Backstory: When I was first suggested homeopathy as an option, I was insulted. I thought it was more of a hospice type of thing for the ones who were not going to get better no matter what. But when I realized it was about wave canceling, it clicked! It made total sense to me. Let's press on.

BTW: It also didn't hurt that it stopped my declining health free fall.

4. I was also positive about how like waves canceled each other. I remember studying this in my math classes in high school, but I also remembered the catch. The waves had to be an EXACT match. Close did not count.

So, since homeopathy worked for me a little, but I couldn't take them anymore, I figured I'd just start holding them. I don't know why I did this. Maybe it was because of an experience I had earlier. This machine at my homeopathic doctor's place said I needed a particular remedy. But when I'd take it, it wouldn't work. It would be too strong for me. She suggested I try holding it instead. Give my body time to adjust to it so I could start taking it. I never would have guessed holding it was where the magic was happening.

Choosing My Starting Point

In one of the NAET (Nambudripad's Allergy Elimination Technique) books from Devi S. Nambudripad, MD, there was a hierarchy list she used.[30] Number one was BBF (autonomic nervous system balance). I didn't know anything about it, nor how to get my hands on it. So, I started with number two: egg. Before Hell Week, I tried her NAET method with practitioners twice and it didn't work. She has huge success with it, and I would recommend her way over mine. However, for me, I didn't have a choice.

Focusing on the concept of canceling a wave, I thought if I could just get egg to "cancel" by itself, everywhere, I might be on to something. I muscle tested to figure out the hierarchy of the meridians in relation to egg. I started with the strongest meridian; the meridian least affected by egg. I did a procedure to neutralize egg during the time of the day for that meridian. It took about twenty minutes. I repeated this procedure when the second strongest meridian time frame appeared. And so on and so forth. It seemed like after each successive meridian was neutralized of egg, the body became stronger. Those stronger meridians helped out the other weaker meridians for egg. It took a few days, but by the time the last three meridians' turn came around, I didn't need to do the procedure for them. It was automatic.

Unbeknownst to me, THAT opened Pandora's box. My body was ready to fight, and fight it did. My body wanted to

---

[30] Nambudripad, Devi S., MD, DC, Lac, PhD (Acu). *NAET: Say Good-Bye to Your Allergies: A Revolutionary Treatment for Allergies and Allergy-Related Conditions* (Delta Publishing Company, 2003), 107.

be well. I could feel a violent tug-of-war going on inside of me. The body wanted to fight egg with other combinations now. It just went on from there. It was interesting how egg affected me so much. I hadn't eaten it for over three years at this point.

I spent the next five years searching for patterns, doing what worked, and not knowing why. While I was continually looking for a perfect wave match, I came up with possibilities of why what I did worked. I would act on them and adjust and still not know why I was so sensitive to everything. Until one day I had the aha moment (Chapters 4 & 5), and all the pieces fell into place. It all made sense. I now knew the enemy: a broken DISH. Now I needed to focus on fixing it.

The Answer

After abandoning the ship of all the known information about our health and our bodies, I decided to crawl back on board with this different perspective in mind. My new information complemented what was already known. It didn't contradict it. It illuminated it. It enabled me to see progress. What they suggested in the past for me would now work.

This gave me hope.

Topic 3: We Have it Backwards

Sometimes, my symptoms were so outlandish, I hesitated to share them because I didn't want to be considered crazy. For example, on one occasion I was taking a shower and my body decided to not inhale again. There was no gasping; there was no noise. There was just no follow-through from exhale. It lasted for about 30 seconds to a minute until I said in my mind very loudly, *Breathe*. It triggered an inhale. How does a body forget to do something like that! So, to me, it wasn't an unrealistic fear that my body would not do what it was supposed to do when it should do it. I knew something big was going on even if it couldn't be seen.

Sometimes, the absence of not being able to prove something wasn't so, was the only way to prove it was. Each level I went up when experimenting on myself, I would sway test what to do next. I would have to assume my answer to my sway test was correct. I would act on those assumptions. If they worked, I would then do the research to try to understand why it did. It felt like I was delving into a science fiction novel because there was no other way to explain it. I believed my body wanted to be well and it had to tell me the answer. I just needed to be willing to listen closely.

I gradually found predictable patterns. I knew what I was doing worked. Going back to very basic science, I am guessing why it worked. By assuming I was right and acting on the presumptions I made, my health improved. It has improved significantly. I have gone through the back door to uncover many things from a different perspective.

Unseen... Is it Invisible?

The old saying "seeing is believing" isn't necessarily all it's cracked up to be. For example, did you know that in America, they were vaccinating for smallpox from 1800?[31] However, the virus was not seen until the invention of the electron microscope 130 years later.[32] Another example is William Harvey. He's known as the man who discovered blood capillaries. He proposed the theory of blood capillaries based on what he observed, even though he could not see the blood capillaries themselves. His fellow comrades scoffed at him and considered him crazy.[33]

Well, what I'm about to share with you will require an open mind. It is just like those examples I've mentioned. They acted on what could not be seen, and eventually science caught up to prove their hypotheses to be accurate. What I'm about to share cannot be seen completely—yet. And maybe it never will be. We still can't SEE gravity. We have to know our enemy before we can beat our enemy. I would like to introduce you to what I believe our real enemy is. I have cut a very rough road to point to the path. The scientists and research doctors can help build this trail into a highway if they

---

[31] Mayo Clinic. "History of Smallpox: Outbreaks and Vaccine Timeline." Mayo Foundation for Medical Education and Research. Last accessed 25 March 2023. https://www.mayoclinic.org/coronavirus-covid-19/history-disease-outbreaks-vaccine-timeline/smallpox.

[32] LibreTexts Biology. "7.10: Discovery and Origin of Viruses." LibreTexts. Last Updated 5 March 2021. https://bio.libretexts.org.

[33] Gregory, Andrew. "William Harvey, English Physician." Britannica. 30 May 2022. https://www.britannica.com/biography/William-Harvey.

so choose. I believe we would all benefit by having this information fine-tuned even more. We could utilize this information to get our nation to stop being so sick.

New Look at Autoimmune Disease

There are more than a hundred disorders falling under the category of autoimmune disease, but they all have one thing in common: the body's immune system is attacking its own tissue and cells. Are all those different disorders obstructing our view of the problem?

Our immune system's job is to protect the body. Protect it against disease or other potentially damaging foreign or abnormal cells. The way the immune system does this is by making antibodies. But... it is making antibodies against itself. Why?

It has been documented over and over that when a person has an autoimmune disease, their body's immune system is attacking its own tissue and cells. When this attacking occurs, it causes chronic inflammation. This, more than usual inflammation, is the cause of the symptoms associated with autoimmune diseases. So, the target for treating the symptoms has been immune-suppressing drugs and similar methods to try to reduce this inflammation.

When I researched autoimmune diseases, two factors always seemed to surface: a trigger and a predisposition for the illness. We are told when these two things are combined, *somehow* the immune system malfunctions. So, we search for the triggers. We search for the genetic factor. We empathize with people stuck in this category.

But...

- What if... the body is in fact protecting itself the only way it knows how?
- What if... it is NOT malfunctioning at all?
- What if... it is just the opposite?
- What if... our immune system has not gone awry?
- We believe the body is malfunctioning and attacking itself, therefore causing inflammation that weakens our immune system.
- What if... it is just the opposite?
- What if... the body is causing inflammation to slow down the immune response because the body is attacking itself?
- Is that a game changer?

What if the body was actually performing what we coin intelligent disobedience?

Intelligent *Disobedience*: "Intelligent disobedience occurs where a service animal trained to help a disabled person goes *directly* against the owner's instructions in an effort to make a better decision."[34]

- *What if...* we assumed the immune system was in fact doing its number one job—protecting the body?
- *What if...* the body was acting under intelligent disobedience?

---

[34] Wikipedia: The Free Encyclopedia. "Intelligent Disobedience." Wikipedia. Last edited 19 July 2022. https://en.wikipedia.org/wiki/Intelligent_disobedience.

- *What if...* inflammation (which slows the immune system down) was the only way the body knew how to protect itself under the given conditions it was in?
- *Would a better question be,* why does the immune system think it needs to slow down?

By switching the cause and effect, EVERYTHING CHANGES. What if inflammation is the body performing intelligent disobedience? We have been looking for WHAT triggered this reaction.

We are trying to find the trigger in SO MANY disorders. Will we be looking forever?

- *What if...* it is not the trigger that matters?
- *What if...* it is just the trigger happening?
- *What if...* the trigger is not one thing?
- *What if...* it is just the straw that broke the camel's back?

And that straw (trigger) can be different for different people and different disorders.

The flipping of the switch is the problem, not the trigger.

As I mentioned before, the list of commonly suspected autoimmune disease factors (triggers to the switch):

- Industrialized countries
- Genetics
- Environment
- Infectious agents
- Hormones
- Viruses (especially Epstein Barr)

- "**Something**" **happened**, and the body is **now attacking itself**.

The trigger could be anything. It's not the triggering agent but the act of being triggered. Getting rid of the trigger is not enough: reducing the load on the camel's back is not enough. This has been tried.

So, the two helpful questions we should ask are...

1. **What happened when the switch was flipped?**
2. **Can it be un-flipped?**

Incidentally, what I discovered would explain the hormone/virus connection, how I am fixing it, and how it fixed me.

What Happened

Let's take a look at the three components associated with autoimmune disease. Let's also assume for a moment the body has an invisible sorting system we are not currently aware of.

A. The Trigger

The trigger flipped a switch. When this switch was flipped, this sorting system became backed up. The body could not keep up with dealing with damaging foreign cells. It may be because the body was already working on other foreign cells (environment, virus, bacteria, parasite, etc.) we may not have been aware of at the time. So, this trigger (whatever it may have been) was the final straw, so to speak. The immune system could no longer keep up. The switch gets flipped.

B. The Predisposition

The predisposition would be a faulty sorting system. If this sorting system had too much to do, it would not be able to keep up. The sorting system would fall behind. So, in order to keep doing its job, it started grouping foreign cells together to try to "catch up." In this process, for example, maybe I drank some orange juice to boost my immune system to fight my virus. Well, if this sorting system was malfunctioning, the nutrients in the orange juice became "grouped" with this virus. So now, when my body encountered this virus, it also encountered the nutrients. However, it now "saw" the nutrients as harmful. So, it started rejecting the nutrients with the virus.

C. The Inflammation

The tug-of-war contest begins. The body is rejecting these nutrients, but the body needs them. The body starts to run low on these nutrients because of rejecting them over a long period of time. Enter inflammation. Inflammation will slow down the immune system. This slowing down will enable the body to hold onto some of the nutrients it desperately needs. It knows it cannot run on empty.

When I first realized this MIGHT be what was going on, I thought the solution would be to just take more supplements. Whatever supplement I was losing, just take LOTS of it.

No. That did not work.

The "wrong" programming was still circulating throughout my body. I needed to stop the errant information. Was that even possible? I found out the answer to that question was YES!

The trigger doesn't matter as much as

knowing the switch has been flipped.

Personal Examples

As I mentioned earlier, my pituitary gland was not working properly. At one point, my acupuncturist said my body was no longer rebuilding itself. This was during the same time I was giving myself human growth hormone shots four times a week. Forcing the pituitary gland to work by taking this medication created the snowball effect of food and environmental allergies. (In case you're wondering, I was at my doctor-determined ideal weight.) My body was powering down and I was trying to force it to power back up. Reflecting on this past experience, I started to ask different questions.

Metabolism Backwards

In the book *The Ultimate Guide to Methylene Blue* by Mark Sloan, he referred to dysfunctional metabolism. He stated that "over ninety percent of diseases that exist today are metabolic in nature. In other words, no disease pathology can be looked at independently from metabolism."[35] But is this causation or correlation?

---

[35] Sloan, Mark. *The Ultimate Guide to Methylene Blue* (Endalldisease Publishing, 2021), 8.

- What if... metabolism wasn't the problem?
- What if... we have it backwards?
- What if... the metabolism problem is because there is a problem?
- What if... it is because the body is powering down to protect itself?
- What if... the body needs to sort before it can power up?
- What if... once the body starts sorting again, the metabolism corrects on its own?

If we factor in a faulty sorting system, could this be a possibility? I'm just asking a loaded question. When I was boosting my metabolism by taking the prescribed human growth hormone shots, I gained new allergies daily. I now believe this was because my body wasn't sorting. Years later, when I was at my naturopath and he told me I needed to boost my metabolism, I was very firm in not taking that route. I explained my reasons and suggested he keep looking. Sure enough, we found the real problem. When it was found, the metabolism quickly and automatically corrected before even leaving his office. Fixing the sorting always fixed my metabolism.

Candida Backwards

I was on a candida diet regiment for I think three years. It was easy not to cheat on it because of the severe ramifications that resulted from doing so. Ugh. According to the book *Candida* by Luc De Schepper, MD, all forms of chronic candidiasis are deficient in magnesium, essential fatty acids, vitamin B6, and a variety of other nutrients.[36]

- What if... I already was avoiding what I was supposed to avoid and taking the extra supplements to boost the nutrient deficiency?
- What if... I was doing this for years and the candida still wasn't subsiding?
- What if... the deficiency is not from diet, but from something else?
- What if... this candida was a way for the body to slow itself down, to protect itself, because something was going on we didn't see?
- What if... this invisible sorting system was malfunctioning?
- What if... the candida was because the body was losing these nutrients from faulty sorting, not from lack of consumption?
- What if... the body was trying to slow down this loss from happening?

Clearing the Bowels Backwards

Have you ever been constipated? Yep. Have you ever taken supplements to aid you in the process? Yep. Have they ever not worked? Yep.

I eventually discovered that when this was happening for me, my body was trying to protect itself. If I had a bowel movement, my immune system would get a boost. Doing this,

---

[36] De Schepper, Luc MD, PhD, CA. *Candida*. (Sante Fe, NM: Full of Life Publishing, 1990), 79.

would cause my nutrient levels to drop too much. What? Therefore, if there was a way to not lose nutrients to faulty sorting, the constipation would go away. From trial and error, I learned that if I held those same supplements where the transverse large intestine was located in my body, thirty minutes of doing this usually gave results within twenty-four hours! FYI: sometimes these supplements were mineral. Metal toxicity is known to cause constipation. Are these minerals and metals somehow connected? I think yes.

Detoxing Backwards

On more than one occasion, my body would be removing harmful Bad Guys very quickly. At one point, I could smell burning nightly during my kidney meridian clock. When we think of burning, we think of acid burns. This isn't always the case. If I look at a pH-level line, the closer to the middle it was (#7) the more neutral it was. Either end was bad. Either end burned.[37] Something very base can burn just as bad as something very acidic. Whatever my body was doing, it was exposing something very base. Processing out too many Bad Guys was burning me? It made no sense. Not sure, I experimented. I realized I needed to cancel the base with an acid instead of just binding it. It helped.

Interestingly, what was causing me to detox so quickly was not from any detox methods. It was from what I share in this book. I just opened the door to let my body do its sorting job.

---

[37] Dock, Elly. "Chemical Burns." Healthline. Updated 20 February 2020. https://www.healthline.com/health/chemical-burn-or-reaction.

What if… there was a way to detox without all the side effects from loss of nutrients? I don't think that is exactly the correct question.

I think a more accurate question would be: if we make it to where the body does not lose these nutrients, can the body detox as quickly as it wants? Or in my case even faster?

Thought to Ponder

- If we assumed the body wanted to be well and everything it did was to accomplish this end result, would the questions change?
- If the body attacking itself is the lesser of the two evils, what is the real evil?
- Is it possible we are in a "what came first, chicken vs. egg" scenario when it comes to our health?
- My ______ organ is causing me problems.
    - Am I deficient in the Good Guys this organ desires?
    - Did this organ malfunction because of the lack of Good Guys or did the organ malfunctioning cause the lack of Good Guys?
- What if inflammation wasn't the problem but it was just a check engine warning light?
- Should we really be disconnecting those wires indicating something isn't working properly?
- What if there was one thing missing from the equation to determine if a person was able to become well or not?
- Could this missing piece be found?
- Could this found piece be fixed?

Conclusion for Chapter 3

I believe looking at the same information from a different angle changed everything. It brought rise to different questions. We saw the inflammation. We saw the problems it caused. We assume it started with the inflammation. Looking back further than the inflammation gave me a different starting point. It gave me different options to visit. It caused me to assume the body was doing what it was meant to do—protect itself. It was just doing it the only way it knew how. What was it protecting itself from? Notice how the different vantage point pointed at different questions. Now I was getting onto a different path. Different questions produced different answers.

Assuming this system was there was one thing. Understanding the way it was causing problems to my health was another. It was believable. How it worked, or how it even got there in the first place, were entirely different questions. But, hey, at least I now knew my enemy. All I needed to do was study the enemy in order to figure out how to beat it.

Section 2

What I Have Learned
About This
Invisible System

CHAPTER 4:
INVISIBLE SYSTEM AT WORK

What I have learned about this possible system.

Opening Story: How I Discovered the Connection (Part One)

I have a nice cup of coffee every morning to start my day. Some call it an addiction. Some would call it a habit or necessary evil. I prefer to think of it as a small pleasure that helps kick-start my day. I was never a coffee drinker until I was in my late 20s. Even then, it was more of a discomfort Band-Aid to make it through the day, and I could only stomach one cup. As time went on, I grew to like the taste of it. Not just the taste of it, but more like the experience of it. On a cold winter morning in Montana, there's just something about waking up slowly to the sound of the coffeepot brewing. Okay, if I get out of bed and dress quickly, the chill that always manages to sneak in through the night will be abated with my warm sweatshirt and my hands wrapped around a warm cup of coffee.

I don't take this small pleasure for granted. For over two years, I was unable to drink coffee. I was unable to eat or drink almost everything. I was severely allergic to so many things. So, this cup of coffee represented progress in my health, and a reminder to enjoy the simple things because I never knew what tomorrow would bring.

Well, this particular morning, I didn't awake to the sound of coffee brewing. I must've forgotten to preset it. Great, I hate it when I do that. So I get dressed and stroll into the kitchen regretting I have to wait ten minutes for my first cup. A whole ten minutes. Silly, right? But guess what? I did have it set. It was just broken. No, anything but that! You would think living out in almost the middle of nowhere, I would have a backup coffeepot. But no, I always put it on the bottom of my priority list. I had to wait until the local store opened. But when they finally opened, they didn't have one! If I drove to the next nearest town, it would have been more than an hour's journey. No, my kids' school needed to take precedence over my cup of coffee.

But as the day wore on, my son thought it would be neat to try to make coffee from scratch. I guess coffeepots didn't always exist. And when we did make camp coffee, we didn't use a pot. But I just didn't like the grinds floating around in my cup afterwards. So, I thought, *let's do it both ways. We will cook the coffee on the stove like we would do over the fire pit when camping*. We thought we were being smart when we decided to filter the brewed coffee through a coffee filter. We placed the coffee filter in a metal strainer. We figured all we had to do was pour the coffee through and we would have ground-free coffee. Big mistake!

Now we know why it takes ten minutes for the coffee to brew. Trying to rush the brewing process only caused a backup and almost total blockage of the flow of water through the filter. What normally took twelve minutes took over thirty when we poured the water too quickly.

Fascinating. It got me thinking. What if this is what is happening with our lymphatic system? What if either the detox organs weren't working properly, or they have too much to work on and this happened? What could that mean?

Overview

We can't see gravity but we know it is there because of what it does. We can't see electrons either, but we have learned so much about them just by studying reactions to tests we do. These tests are how we discovered electrons rotate around protons. I am suggesting our invisible system is there based on what happened when I assumed it was.

For this invisible system, I would like for you to imagine we have an invisible shield around us. I have called it the Defensive Individual Shield Hypothesis (DISH). This shield (DISH) has two jobs. The malfunctioning of this shield was the root cause of my problems. How did I come up with this acronym, and what does it mean? Let me break it down for you.

The Invisible System Summarized

Defensive: The First Job of Protecting the Body

I believe this shield has two jobs. Its first job is protecting the body. It is defending us against the environment we are exposed to on a daily basis. We cannot see this shield, just like we can't see atoms. We forget atoms are even there. Everything is made up of atoms and all atoms are made up of protons, neutrons, and electrons. (Hydrogen has no neutrons.) The electrons spin around their nucleus, and these electrons give off energy. This energy, in turn, acts almost like a tiny force field. This tiny force field is protecting us. I will go into more detail about this when we get to the S part of this acronym.

Individual: Unique for Each Person

I know there is talk of chakras and a universal energy force. I don't know anything about that. I am talking about *just* individual shields existing around a person's immediate body based on what they allow into their body. These are individualized for each person. I believe the sweat, bacteria, and excess lymph continually on the surface of a person's skin has a type of frequency to it. This "frequency" varies throughout the day based on what has "made its way" to the surface of the individual's skin. This frequency changing is what helps the DISH to do its second job—sorting.

Shield: It's a Frequency Barrier for Sorting—Job Two

This energy field surrounding our body, I have called a shield. I believe it is an electrical and/or magnetic field creating a protective barrier with a frequency to it. I believe the frequency it creates enables our body to do the sorting job I've been talking about. The defensive protective coating I mentioned earlier from those atoms is not only preventing weaker frequencies from entering our body by deflecting them, but also sorting the ones leaving the body as well.

Hypothesis: It's an Idea

According to merriam-webster.com, a hypothesis is "an idea that is proposed for the sake of argument so that it can be tested to see if it might be true." So, I'm not saying I know it all and this is how it is OR that it is definitely true, but what I am saying is that there is something to this. There is enough here to look deeper. Otherwise, **how could holding the supplements and remedies be more effective than taking them**?

I decided to assume DISH was true. In the beginning, I assumed the problem was DISH failing to properly do its first job—protecting. I had not grasped the concept of its second job yet. I started to base all my decisions for my health on this shield; my health held. I stopped the free fall.

Later, when I started visiting the idea of this shield's second job of assisting me in sorting out all the environmental things I encountered every day, my health improved! The sorting idea was originally meant for when there was a co-infection. It was meant to tackle one challenge at a time. But, over the years and through trial and error, I came to discover it was much more than that. Was it some rare fluke that I just magically got better as I understood the depths of what I was figuring out? *I really don't think so.*

Topic 1: DISH's First Job

The first job of my DISH was to create an energy field. This field prevented the body from having two things combine with each other on an energy level. For example, think of frequencies as different colors. Let's say red was in my body. I came into contact with yellow in my environment. This shield would prevent the red and yellow from making orange. This would in turn make it where the body only needed to remove red. Not only did the shield prevent yellow from entering, but orange would also be a nonissue. It was unable to be formed.

How This Is Accomplished

Let's start with—everything has energy and therefore has magnetism. I looked at the definitions of energy and magnetism to see if, indeed, we could possibly have a field around us. If so, what could that mean?

Everything is made of energy.

This is such common knowledge that we had hammered into our heads in school science classes that sometimes we don't even see it when it's right in front of our eyes. Atoms do not have to get energy from somewhere, because they are energy. And since everything is made up of atoms, everything has energy.

Einstein even proposed that mass and energy are two sides of the same coin.[38] Mass can convert into energy and

---

[38] Perkowitz, Sidney. "E=mc^2." Britannica. Date unknown. https://www.britannica.com/science/E-mc2-equation.

vice-versa. In reality, that would mean all matter we see is a manifestation of energy.

Matter is nothing but hyper-condensed energy, and this energy can vibrate at different frequencies, giving rise to fundamental forces based on the vibrational patterns.

Everything has magnetism too.

According to livescience.com, "The motion of electrically charged particles gives rise to magnetism... all materials experience magnetism, some more strongly than others."[39]

We are made up of atoms. Atoms are energy. Atoms are electrically charged particles; therefore, they have some magnetism.

DISH is a possible magnetic field.

In *The Geology Book* by Dr. John D. Morris, it states, "The invisible magnetic field around the earth is a result of the earth having an iron core, in much the same way that an iron bar magnet produces a magnetic field."[40] We need iron in our blood to live. Maybe, just maybe, we have, so to speak, an iron core.

Dr. Morris goes on to say that, "Even though we only know about them from theory, it does appear that electrical currents flowing in the outer core's conductive metal generate the earth's magnetic field. **This is extremely**

---

[39] Sutter, Paul, and Jim Lucas. "What Is Magnetism? Facts About Magnetic Fields and Magnetic Force." Livescience. Last accessed 22 June 2020. https://www.livescience.com/38059-magnetism.html.

[40] Morris, Dr. John D. *The Geology Book* (Master Books, 2000), 7.

important because the magnetic field shields the earth [emphasis added] from harmful radiation coming from the sun and stars. Without it, life would be completely impossible on planet earth."[41]

So, this magnetic field protects the earth by causing rays from the sun to deflect off of it. On a smaller scale, would having an energy field around me help protect me from being bombarded by harmful things as well? A type of force field, so to speak?

This would be Job One of a properly working DISH**. This magnetic field** would deflect or repel weaker energy fields than the one we are giving off. Remember, everything has energy. Everything we come into contact with every day has energy. When this repelling fails to happen, the body is compromised. We are only able to repel the energy fields that are weaker than our own.

It was like the card game War. The highest card won. The strongest energy field won. If my body failed at this repelling, the stronger energy field had the potential of combining with what was weakening my body in the first place—what my body was focusing on at that time. It is possible that when this happened, energy fields became combined. What does that even mean? Well, this means (using colors as an example), if red and yellow are together, the problem just became more complicated because now I have orange as well.

[41] Morris, *The Geology Book*, 8.

The idea that electrons circulating around an object is enough to prevent other objects from coming into contact with it may seem a little strange. There is a video on YouTube that demonstrates this very thing with copper and a magnet. The video is published by NightHawkInLight. It is called "Copper's Surprising Reaction to Strong Magnets | Force Field Motion Dampening."[42] Check it out. It is a very fascinating video.

For now, here is an example of what it looks like on a typical day.

A Cup of Coffee

Let's look again at my cup of coffee. Is it really just a cup of coffee? Energy cannot be created or destroyed. So what is the cup of coffee really?

I pour myself a cup of black coffee. (I'll keep it simple.) So far, so good. I am stronger than anything I have come into contact with. The coffeepot's water tank and filter holder were made of plastic and possibly went through a metal or paper filter. Some non-drip pots have metal coils the coffee drips over to get to the glass or metal pot. Another energy field.

This isn't even including the cushion of the chair I'm about to sit on. What about the legs of the chair? Are they the same material? How about the table I plan to set my coffee cup on? What is the tabletop made of?

---

[42] NightHawkInLight. *"Copper's Surprising Reaction to Strong Magnets | Force Field Motion Dampening." (00:07:45) 26 January 2018. Online Video Clip. YouTube.* https://youtu.be/sENgdSF8ppA.

What did I pour the coffee into? Ceramic? Porcelain? Plastic? Metal? Did I touch a metal cabinet knob to open the cupboard door to get my cup out? Is the cabinet door painted? All of these objects have energy fields that are bouncing off my energy field. I have the stronger field.

What if something was weakening my DISH? What if I had the computer or radio on or my cell phone in my pocket?

What if I touched the light switch to turn the light on? Or I walked by the refrigerator when it kicked on? All of those have a much stronger energy field than all the other previous items I mentioned. They might even have a stronger energy field than me. For me, that is all it took for the difference between "shields up" or "shields down."

Energy fields staying separate and energy fields mixing with each other. If this was what was happening, oh man! I was overwhelmed at first. Do you realize how many possible combinations of mixed energy fields there could be? I was a math major and I don't even want to figure out the answer. An incomprehensible number!

Just my body having a shield to protect itself would enable me to better utilize the nutrients and hormones I had. This would require less effort and work on my detox organs. Having this full tank to draw from enabled me to be healthy. Healthy people produce wider energy fields around their bodies. This requires anything trying to attack the body to have to work harder to penetrate through this shield.

Something to Think About

Before I share this next part, I want to start off by saying, a big part of science is observation—even if we aren't even sure of what we are observing or how to test it. Some may suggest I saw more than what was there, but by observing this, I believe I was observing the first job of DISH.

My observation...

Have you ever noticed when you are outside in the summer with a group of friends or family and there are mosquitoes or flies buzzing about that, for most people, are just a nuisance, but for others, they look like they have a banquet sign hanging around their neck? It isn't their imagination. It's almost like they have an attractant on them.

For example, one family camping trip we were on, the mosquitoes were particularly bad. But they were also visibly biased. Some people had none of them landing on them; they were just hovering and being a nuisance. Some may have one or two occasionally land on them. Then there is always the person who the mosquitoes love! Well, one evening we arrived in the woods, parked the trailer, and all the excited kids poured out of the vehicle. One son always needed the bug repellant first. Before I could even get the can out of the car, he probably had 20 mosquitoes on his legs, arms, and back. I now wonder if it was because his DISH was broken. (He did have health problems.) Did the rest of the family have strong DISHes preventing the mosquitoes from landing?

Another example, years later I noticed a similar situation when I needed to be outside for a batch neutralizing session. (This will be explained in section three of this book.) I needed to be away from electricity to be the strongest energy field. I know this will be hard to understand, but after a few years of being very aware of my DISH, I was able to instinctively tell when it was up or down/low. Well, this particular day, I had my leg stretched out to place a few drops on my leg. A fly came by to keep me company. He landed on my leg. When my shield went up, he flew off my leg and hovered around it. The second I felt my shield go down again the fly landed. This continued for almost ten minutes! Over and over again. Very interesting. Once my batch was done and my shield stayed up, it hovered for a while and then left. Coincidence?

Topic 2: DISH's Second Job

The second job of DISH lightens the load the body needs to process. It lightens the load by adjusting frequencies on the surface of the skin to enable the body to do its sorting job better. It allows the body to deal with one challenge at a time. How does this sorting occur?

The Coating Giving Off This Frequency

Where does this frequency come from? There is a "coating" on our skin. Even when it appears clean, there are things on the surface of our skin. We have bacteria, sweat, and excess lymph continually present there.

What is the reason for them being there? Could these things be creating a frequency beneficial to the body?

1. Healthy skin has bacteria on it.

May 28, 2009

> *Your skin is crawling with hundreds of kinds of bacteria, NIH researchers find. There are up to a hundred times more kinds of bacteria thriving in "vibrant communities" on healthy skin than previously known, report NIH researcher Elizabeth A. Grice, PhD, and colleagues at the National Human Genome Research Institute.*[43]

---

[43] DeNoon, Daniel J. "Human Skin Alive with Bacteria: Skin Crawls with Many More 'Vibrant Communities' of Bacteria Than Thought." WebMD. 28 May, 2009. https://www.webmd.com/skin-problems-and-treatments/news/20090528/human-skin-alive-with-bacteria#1.

2. We sweat. There are almost no Bad Guys in sweat.

We hear about the need to exercise and sweat so we can remove toxins from our bodies. Apparently, this is not accomplished by quantity. I found this on the internet.

> *At most, Imbeault and his colleagues found, a typical person doing 45 minutes of high-intensity exercise a day could sweat a total of two liters a day—normal background perspiration included—and all that sweat would contain less than one-tenth of a nanogram of these pollutants.*[44]

Looking at this sweat, the results of removing toxins are minuscule.

Allow me to help you with the math. A nanogram is one billionth of a gram and that gram would need to be cut into ten pieces. Only one of those pieces would contain toxins. TINY amount! But...it is present on the surface of the skin. Is its presence, regardless of how small, just enough to change the frequency of this coating I am talking about?

3. Excess fluid (lymph) goes to the surface of the skin.

Our kidneys and liver filter our blood and the lymphatic system grabs up Bad Guys in the body to enable the body to fight those foreign bodies. The excess lymph then exits the body through the skin.

---

[44] National Geographic Society. "Fact or Fiction: Can You Really Sweat Out Toxins?" National Geographic. 6 April 2018. https://www.nationalgeographic.com/science/article/sweating-toxins-myth-detox-facts-saunas-pollutants-science.

What can affect the lymphatic system? What can cause this DISH to break?

- Viruses
- Bacteria
- Blockage
- Parasites
- Radiation
- Surgery

Other Scientific Information I Needed to Know

1. *Everything has energy.* Energy consists of frequency and amplitude. Therefore, everything has frequency. If everything has frequency, then this coating also has a frequency.

2. *Another accepted fact is that like waves cancel.* (The scientific name for this is destructive interference.) However, in order for this to happen, the waves have to be the same.

3. *Energy fields have been observed around people in laboratory tests.* They range from two inches to six feet. There appears to be a connection between the size of the energy field and the health of the individual. Healthy people have larger ranges while unhealthy people have smaller ranges. These smaller ranges are usually accompanied by gaps as well.[45]

---

[45] Korotkov, K. "Measuring Human Energy Field Revolutionary Instrument to Reveal Energy Fields of Human and Nature." Semantic Scholar. 2012. https://www.semanticscholar.org/paper/Measuring-Human-Energy-Field-Revolutionary-to-of-Korotkov/531ce58e34aca26a7ca9ae812b60cac0ec2e0865.

What This Frequency Is Doing

We are going to start off with a math lesson. We have the coating, we have the skin, and we have the stuff in the body that needs to leave. We have ourselves a primitive math equation. Look at it like it is an algebra problem. The skin is the equal sign. If something is on the inside of the body and on the surface of the skin, the body just lets it leave. They cancel each other. They are the same. Their frequencies are the same. Like waves cancel. The other organs don't have to process it out.

Let's look at the math problem. To make it simple and friendly, instead of using numbers, I'm going to use objects—food in this example. The main point, though, is how we solve the problem. We should always simplify it first whenever possible.

For example, if we have a math problem like this one:

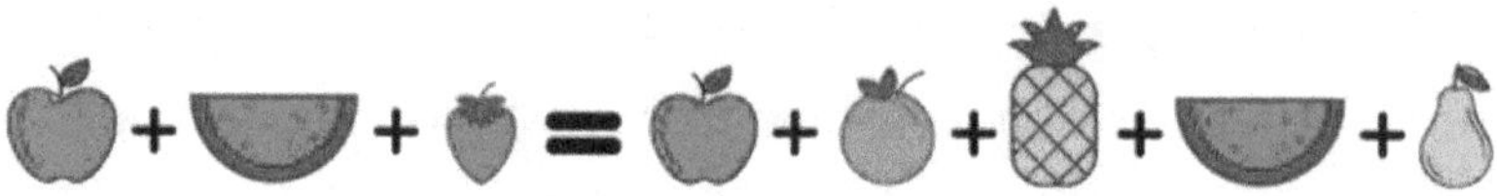

We want to simplify the problem before we get down to the nitty gritty of solving it. We would start off by looking to see if there are any terms (objects) the same on both sides of the equal sign. If there are, they cancel each other out.

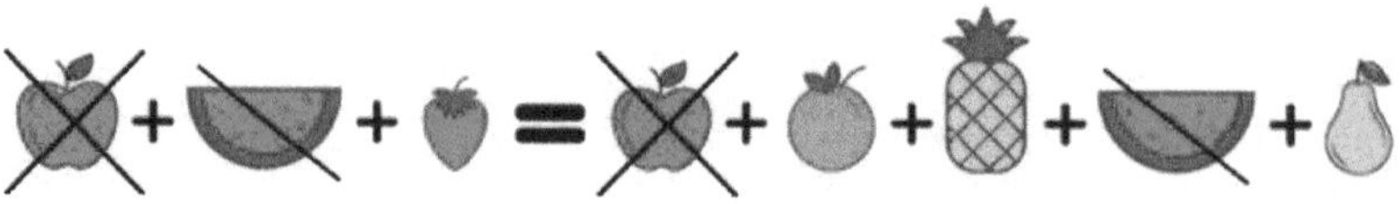

By doing this, we are able to reduce it down to what we need to focus on.

In this example, we would need to make the strawberry frequency be the same as the three other fruits.

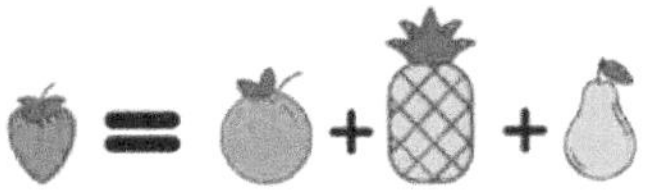

That is basically what I was manually doing for my body! I was manually lightening the load so it could focus on what it needed to. My lymphatic system was unable to do its job. It was failing to adjust the coating on my skin.

The absence of the coating was preventing me from being able to cancel and narrow down what needed to be done. This coating needed to be continually changing based on what I encountered throughout the day.

If the substance was in my body and on my body, they canceled each other. By canceling, the body didn't need to process them. We know healthy people sweat. I know I didn't. I also know I had lymphatic system problems.

Scientists have mentioned there is a connection between the immune system and the lymphatic system. Maybe this DISH is just an expansion on this idea. Maybe understanding DISH would help us to better understand the relationship between these two systems.

What if, when the lymphatic system is overburdened, the excess lymph that usually comes to the surface of the skin is unable to? What if this is what causes the breakdown? This blockage may have caused the switch to be flipped. The sorting system stopped. As a result, more than one thing happened.

1. The body was unable to target one Bad Guy at a time.

2. The Bad Guy may mix with another Bad Guy to make it more difficult to remove.

3. The Good Guy may get mixed with a Bad Guy. (I'll get into more detail about this in the next chapter.)

- Only the Bad Guys are supposed to be grabbed by the system.
- If Good Guys have no place to go, will they get grabbed up too?

Topic 3: DISH Can Be Automatic or Manual

As my health continued to improve, I started noticing things I did not need to do, as well as things I could now do. Let's face it, most techniques and treatments work for most people. I believe these people have a working DISH. If the appropriate protocol wasn't working or they had an allergic reaction to it, maybe it is because the person's DISH is broken.

On Autopilot

When there is no interference and the system is working and sorting as it should, there is no grouping of Good and Bad Guys. When the system encounters more than one Bad Guy and it becomes burdened, it may target one Bad Guy and let the other one get away for now. It has been observed under a microscope how a team of Good Guys may choose to not attack a Bad Guy. It measured up the Bad Guy and then just left. The Bad Guy is left alone. To go where? To the surface of the skin? Maybe. The lymphatic system basically delegates the removing of the second Bad Guy to our skin. (The skin is another detox organ.) Once it is done making the Attacker cells it needs to get rid of the first Bad Guy, it will then focus on the second Bad Guy. The lymph nodes would then start grabbing Bad Guy #2 to create Attacker cells for it. This worked as long as the exit roads stayed open.

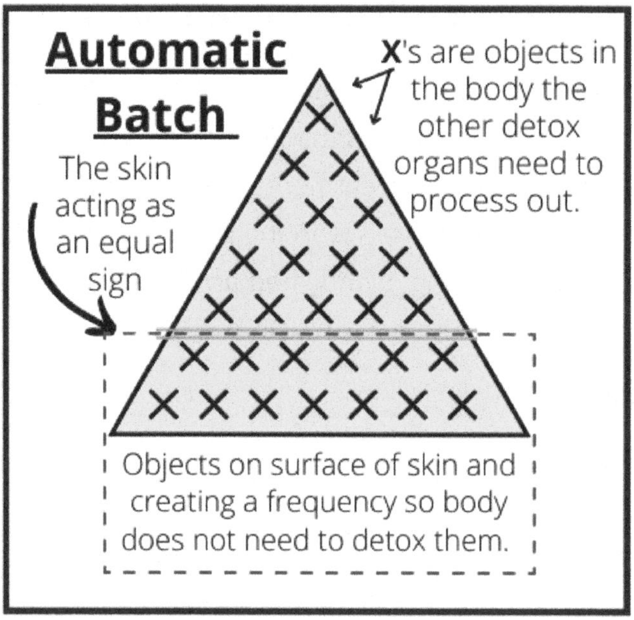

Self-Correcting

If by chance these roads are unable to stay open and grouping of a Good Guy and a Bad Guy occur, the body is able to self-correct. How? By doing the same thing. The information in the system may be off, but if either the Good Guy or the Bad Guy is reintroduced into the system by itself WHILE the DISH is working, it will sort it again and adjust the information. It will identify the Good Guy by himself and let him go. It will continue to remove the Good Guy with the Bad Guy but all the while leaving the solidary Good Guy alone.

But... I suspect this is only possible for heterogeneous batches. Don't worry, we will cover batches in more detail in section three, chapter 8. On the good note, most batches seemed to be this heterogeneous type. I also suspect when it is a heterogeneous batch, the healthful lifestyle is able to correct it. I speculate that when medical recommendations are given and don't work in spite of a properly functioning DISH, it is because homogeneous and/or Mimicker batches are involved. If I have you totally confused, quickly glance at the glossary to see the definitions for these types of batches.

Manual Correcting

By doing this, **I mainly focused on trying to make my outside equal the inside** as much as possible by doing *batches*. This enabled the supplements I had tried before to no avail to now work! I just needed to hold them. Depending on what area of my body was being affected and what type of batch I was dealing with determined how I needed to go about doing this. I occasionally needed to take them as well, but for the most part, a faulty DISH was causing my body to reject nutrients. By holding them, the body stopped rejecting them. The Good Guys had an exit route to avoid being grabbed up.

What does this look like? This is when knowledge of organs, meridians, acupuncture/acupressure points came in handy. What also helped was being able to look up the different uses of different essential oils. In the beginning, what I used most was just the environment around me. At one point, carrying a Lego brick around in my pocket worked wonders for my energy level and how well my lungs worked. Insane, I know. It was the plastic, but not just the plastic. Sometimes it needed to be black, other times white, yellow, or blue. I suspect it is because plastic was present in the list of Camp Lejeune water toxins. Holding it enabled me to work on other Bad Guys instead. A load my body could handle.

With the rejecting ceased, I needed to correct any misinformation or missing information caused by the chain reaction. I will explain this in the next chapter too.

Personal Examples

The Body Trying to Make Its Own DISH

What I found to be fascinating here is my body was attempting to do this long term and short term. I just never really thought to notice it this way before.

Short term: The symptoms that are sometimes accompanied by a virus could be the body trying to place something on the outside of the body because it was being overburdened by a virus. For example, bleeding gums, sweats, or pox. This is something in the body but that is now on the outside of the body, creating a coating for a frequency to be located in. Maybe, when the body does this, it is attempting to separate out two or more components, in order to make the workload on the organs lighter during the trying time of the virus.

Long term: We have all heard the saying "x marks the spot." Well... I have many moles on my body. Whenever I needed to target a particular organ or meridian, guess what? There was almost always a freckle or a mole or a skin tag in the location of where it needed to be. On two separate occasions, before I knew what I now know, I had a mole removed from two different locations. Both times, a flat mole or discoloration of the skin would show up within a few inches from where the mole was removed. This mole, freckle, or skin tag was my body attempting to place something on the outside of the body to aid in this sorting process.

I have included two pictures of my daughter. She was born with no moles on her body. Her moles started showing up when she was eighteen months old. I think this was her body trying to make a temporary DISH for her. The before picture was after the moles had been on her body for several years. Several had fallen off by the time we took the first picture. The second picture was taken a year later. The only thing I ever physically placed on these moles was a Band-Aid when it came to the scabbing stage of falling off. This is when it would be tender, so it was more for padding than anything. Hard to believe. The only thing we did was manually help her

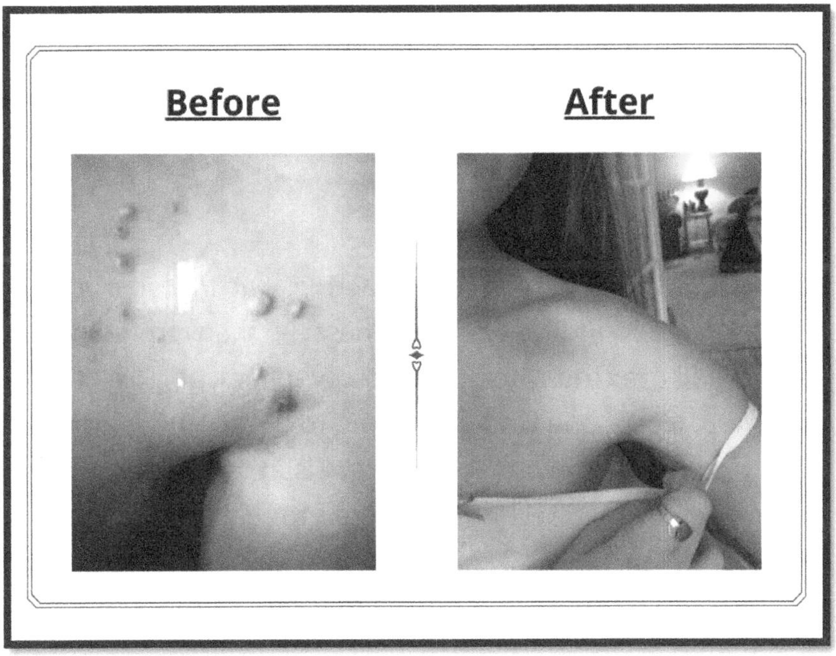

body to do DISH's second job, sorting. When the moles were no longer needed as a DISH, they just fell off. This also happened when a mole appeared and disappeared on my husband's back and arm.

Another possible example: The intestinal flora (good bacteria in the intestines) is key in our immune system. In the book *Clean Gut* by Alejandro Junger, MD, he states beautifully, "Throughout the digestive tube different immune-system 'stations' are located directly on the other side of the intestinal wall, opposite where the good bacteria settle. These good bacteria help keep the immune system in check. The immune system generally attacks bacteria, but **it seems to have a truce with the bacteria of the intestinal flora**, [emphasis added] as long as they don't try to get into the bloodstream."[46]

Do equal signs work on the inside of the body too?

Good question, no answer.

Thought to Ponder

At this point, maybe you're wondering, *but that is a lot of frequencies*. It sounds like one big mess. So many frequencies zooming all over the place. Yes. However, look at it like it is a train yard. Not a lone track pulling up to a station, but a huge train yard, with many, many tracks crisscrossing and trains racing by in every direction. Do I need to feel overwhelmed? No. The only thing I really need to worry about is whether or not there is a train on the same track I was currently on.

---

[46] Junger, Alejandro MD, *Clean Gut: The Breakthrough Plan for Eliminating the Root Cause of Disease and Revolutionizing Your Health* (New York, NY: HarperOne, an Inprint of HarperCollins Publishers, 2013), 40.

You will see this is true when I tell you more about DISH. We will have to isolate this train troublemaker (Bad Guy) in order to fix the problem.

Maybe you are also wondering about this coating I keep talking about. Remember, the coming to the surface of the skin isn't an all-or-nothing exit strategy for the nutrients and hormones our bodies need. On a cellular level, our blood vessels are like soaker hoses. Most of the water (blood) goes from point A to point B. This *water majority* does what it is supposed to do in the organs and throughout the body. Only a small amount does not reach its destination. The small amount is what leaks out and goes to the surface of the skin to create the frequency to allow the body to not reject the rest of the *water* that did get from point A to point B. If it gets redirected, it will go through the lymphatic system and potentially be labeled as a Bad Guy. I have dedicated the next chapter to go into more detail about this.

Manually making a DISH is like CPR. Not ideal, but necessary until the body can do it again itself.

Conclusion for Chapter 4

By acknowledging the possibility of there being two types of people, it changes everything. The type A person has a working DISH and is able to use methods and protocols to improve their health and succeed. The type B person does not, unless she does it manually. Knowing this piece was missing and doing something about it put me back in the game.

It seems when the questions change, everything changes. With the body malfunctioning like this, could drugs fix it or would it just be adding more Bad Guys to the problem? Failing to sort something... and adding more to the something. Is there any way to fix it? Any way to take the something to help me without it adding to the problem. Yes!

We know inflammation has been around for decades. If only there was a reset button. The reset button I tried before did not work. Maybe there was a way to find a different one. I understood holding my supplements usually worked better than taking them. I understood what happened that took me from one side of the *something happened* to the other side of it. But was there a way to get back? Now I was asking the right questions.

In the quest for finding the answers, I learned more about the system and how it significantly affected me more than I could imagine. Understanding how it did operate enabled me to narrow down the many variables that made this simple concept complicated. It helped me to know where to put my focus when it did break. It also helped me to know what to do manually to avoid having it break again.

CHAPTER 5: WHY DISH IS IMPORTANT

Grasping the significance of how DISH affects our health.

Opening Story: How I Discovered the Connection (Part Two)

You may be wondering how on earth did she figure this all out? Short answer: I was desperate and homebound. I had a life-span clock ticking off my last days and those were being spent just lying in bed because I could do nothing else. So, needless to say, I had a very strong motive and lots of time on my hands. Lots of time to think. To think about all the books I had read up to this point. To think about what they were missing and why they didn't work. It wasn't easy. As I mentioned before, I knew like waves canceled. But why was I the only one who seemed to be so sensitive to this concept? It took me five years of doing it manually before I realized why I had to do it. How did I know what to use day by day? Trial and error. Much trial and error, as well as learning to listen to what my body was trying to say.

For example, back to the water fast I told you about in Chapter 2. My body did not reset. But during this time, life had to go on. Kids needed to be fed. Groceries needed to be put away. The hunger was real. But wait, the hunger pangs suddenly disappeared. What did I just do? I had grabbed a lemon to put away. If I was holding the lemon, I didn't feel hungry. Confusing, yes. But I went with it. At one point, my hands were full but I didn't want to put the lemon down. So, I shoved it in my sock. The following day, I noticed I was feeling hungry again. I figured I needed to go back to holding the lemon. I reached down and grabbed it out of my sock. But no, I was in disbelief. That fresh lemon had turned into a brown, hard golf ball in less than 24 hours. I placed a new fresh one in my sock and the hunger was gone. Can I explain why it happened? No. Did I benefit from it? Yes. So, I did it. I filed this information away in the back of my mind for later.

When I started working on eliminating food allergies later, I needed an essential oil to help me. My mind retrieved this prior experience, and I chose to try lemon oil. It worked. Is it the only one that would have worked? I don't know. But if it isn't broke, don't fix it. So I stuck with it until it didn't. The only time it didn't seem to work was when I was working with egg. Hyssop oil worked then. On other occasions I really didn't know what to try, so I would look at what I had and sway test to see if any would work. I noticed if I was dealing with missing information, sometimes I just needed to make the mental connection of what the information was or what oil would work. Other times I would need the item in my energy field. How did I figure that out? Sway testing to figure out what I needed and then once I narrowed it down, I no longer needed it. The missing information being found was always accompanied by a change in my breathing pattern. It could be a cough, sneeze, shortness of breath, yawn, a big inhale, or several very short breaths in quick repetition.

Getting back to my point of how I discovered the second connection, I had had a crazy few days. I had neutralized benzene on myself. It resulted in a slew of parasite die-offs over the next several months. Parasites came out of my body everywhere. Some perforated my skin lengthwise to abandon ship. At this point in my life, we had moved to a lower elevation (from Montana to Texas). I was able to somewhat tolerate the computer. I had about two hours before my entire right arm and hand would go numb and I would develop a headache. But I had those two hours. I spent it researching what was currently happening to me. Growing up, my family and I had been exposed to lymphatic parasites while we were stationed with my dad in Turkey. We all had received one dose of treatment to kill them. Here I was reading it took several doses. I also read they are mostly asymptomatic and cause significant damage to the body before being symptomatic. Interesting.

But why? Why did neutralizing benzene bring this on? Was it just a boost in my immune system or something else? I only received one dose of medicine decades ago for these lymphatic parasites. I started searching for what drug they might have given me. As I was reading, I fell back in my chair in disbelief. Many drugs used to fight parasitic infections contained benzene. Something happened when I copied this benzene wave. But what?

My time was up at the computer. I went back to my bed to rest and hold the jars on my body in particular locations as I had been doing for years. If I did this for twenty minutes every four hours, I could usually go about the rest of my day normally. As I lay there, I was thinking. What was leaving my body sure looked like those parasites. Camp Lejeune caused lymphatic issues as well. Did my problem have something to do with the lymphatic system? Was my lymphatic system broken? Does the lymphatic system do what I had been manually doing? Is the lymphatic system supposed to create the frequency I needed to manually place on myself? I think so! I originally realized it is how my body divided and conquered problems. Only later, through trial and error when I was stuck at a process I couldn't overcome, did I realize I could break it down even further, which led me to realize this did not only include harmful products but beneficial ones as well!

Once I realized what I was manually doing for my body, it took me another five years to learn about the details of it, which I will share with you. When you read this, keep in mind you are reading a summary of over ten years of my life. It took time to figure it out. One time, it took me over nine months to realize one problem. However, while trying to figure it out, I was still able to function based on the concept of creating a manual shield. Once I figured out the piece to the puzzle, though, I was able to move on to more difficult Bad Guys.

Overview

Let's start off with an analogy and then I'll explain in slightly more science-y terms what I believe is happening.

What Is Happening Here?

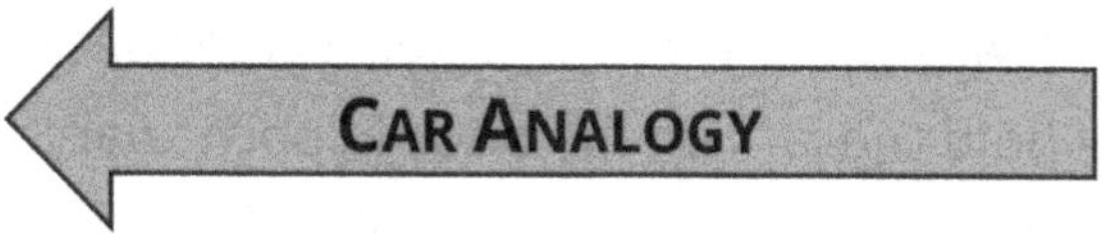

First, picture if you will your circulatory system. More specifically, the end of your circulatory system. This is where the blood capillaries are. These blood capillaries have tiny gaps between their cells that allow fluid, but not blood, to escape the circulatory system. I guess you could kind of look at it like it is a soaker hose. Fluid is flowing through the hose, but it is also leaking out of it all along the way. When this fluid escapes, it needs to go someplace. Generally speaking, it has to either get reabsorbed or exit the body. (This is where the "coating" that makes the frequency on our skin comes from.) Let's say this "soaker hose" is a super road. Let's also pretend this fluid is cars. When these cars leave this super road, they are going onto a busy highway in the middle of a big city. Exit ramps are everywhere. Cars going in every direction.

Now, I would like you to imagine all these cars being different colors. Blue cars, green cars, red cars, and yellow cars. Imagine also these exit ramps. However, in this imaginary world, each ramp is a designated color. These colored cars can only exit at their designated color of ramp. Red cars can only exit the red ramp. Blue cars can only exit the blue ramp, and so on and so forth. If the car does not have a colored ramp corresponding to it, it gets redirected to the lymphatic side road.

There is a traffic guard at the entrance to this side road. His job is to control the amount of traffic entering the side road. He only allows so many cars through at a time.

There is also a rear guard stationed at this same side road. The rear guard's job is to decide if the passengers in these cars are beneficial to the system and allowed to reenter. If the passengers are harmful, they are not allowed to reenter.

Everything runs smoothly until rush hour (a sickness/chemical overburdens the system) or until a ramp becomes blocked (parasites/injury/etc.). Now, more traffic has to be diverted to this "side road." Cars are starting to back up. There is a traffic jam. (The lymph nodes may become swollen.) Now the exit ramps AND side road are both getting backed up. The road system becomes saturated. It can't handle any more. Nobody is going anywhere. Something needs to be done to get the traffic moving again. Damage control begins.

The traffic guard at the entrance to the side road informs the passengers of these cars that only so many vehicles are allowed to pass in a given amount of time. So, some people abandon their vehicles to carpool with other people. It gets the traffic flowing again. But...

The problem here is some Bad Guys might hop into the same car as a Good Guy.

When this car gets to the end of the side road, there is the second guard. This guard shines the flashlight into the car and looks around. He sees the Bad Guy and informs all passengers, good or bad, that this car is not allowed to reenter the system.

The Good Guy must be rejected with the Bad Guy.

However, if the rear guard has been rejecting this type of car for too long, there will be a shortage of Good Guys in the system. This is bad as well. The body MUST have a given number of Good Guys to get the job done. So, what happens? The head office will give an executive order to allow the Bad Guy to reenter the system. He is now one of the Good Guys, but not really. This causes nothing but trouble. But the head office considers it a necessary evil to keep the system running.

So, whether it is the accepting of the Bad Guy or the rejecting of the Good Guy, both are bad news. Both are false information. Either might get programmed into the so-called system now. But to keep it simple, let's just look at when the

Good Guy is the one being rejected. Because the car has been banned (not the passengers), any vehicle matching that description will also be banned. Think of your favorite cop or detective movie—a BOLO (Be on the Lookout) has been made for the car. They don't care who is driving it. This guilt by association has now made the passengers in the car an enemy to the system. The traffic jam, which caused this problem in the first place (the swollen lymph nodes), may go away, but the false information (*mis*information) is still circulating. This particular car is still not allowed to reenter.

The only way the Good Guy will be able to correct this *mis*understanding is by giving the guards some new information. This Good Guy needs to prove he is not associated with this Bad Guy. This is accomplished by making new off-ramps to make the flow of traffic more effective. These Good Guys are then able to avoid the side road. They are able to avoid being forced to stay in their carpool vehicle. They are able to avoid being rejected. The Bad Guy ends up taking the side road by himself and is caught and removed.

So when this saturation occurred, the body was no longer able to adjust these exit ramps to do what was needed to keep the traffic moving. When this "coating" (the adjuster) on my body was missing, the off-ramps were blocked. This caused the traffic jam in the lymphatic system. This in turn caused a breakdown in the sorting system.

Using an example...

For example, my body was unable to separate the bad strontium 90 (Camp Lejeune water poisoning) from the good strontium the body needed to function properly. It was rejecting both! (Is this what is happening with autoimmune diseases?) No matter how much strontium I took, I still did not have enough for my body system to function properly. The good strontium needed to stop being associated with the bad strontium. They needed to be independent of each other. Once I trained my body to recognize the difference between the two types of strontium, taking the strontium supplements brought the levels back up to normal. I then needed to take the supplements only for a short period of time. I now no longer need to take strontium!

How did I make the good strontium independent of the bad strontium? I created a new "off-ramp" for the good strontium to take. By doing this, my body stopped rejecting the good with the bad.

How did I make this new ramp? The very simplified answer was holding good strontium in my energy field. (It was way more complicated than this. There were many other additional factors (Bad Guys) involved to bring this batch to a climax before I could do this step, but do you get the picture? I know there are several holes in this analogy, but it is the best way I can explain this concept for now.

Misinformation Source

The lymphatic system became too crowded.

The Good Guys road becomes blocked.

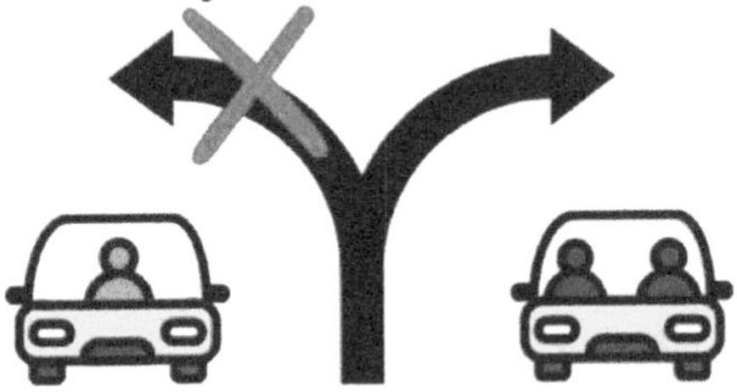

They get redirected and grabbed up with the Bad Guys. Doing this causes them to become combined.

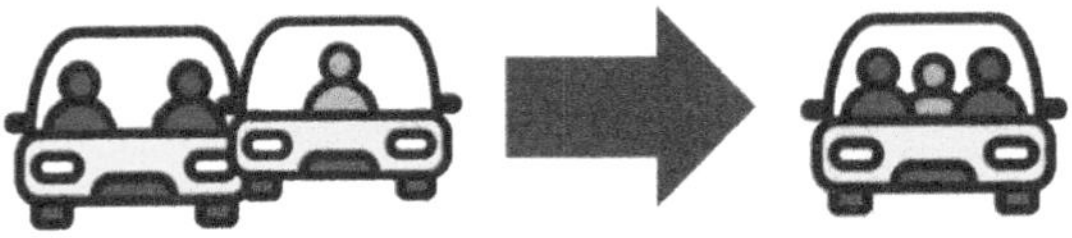

The system keeps rejecting the Good Guys with the Bad Guy. (Body Attacks Itself)

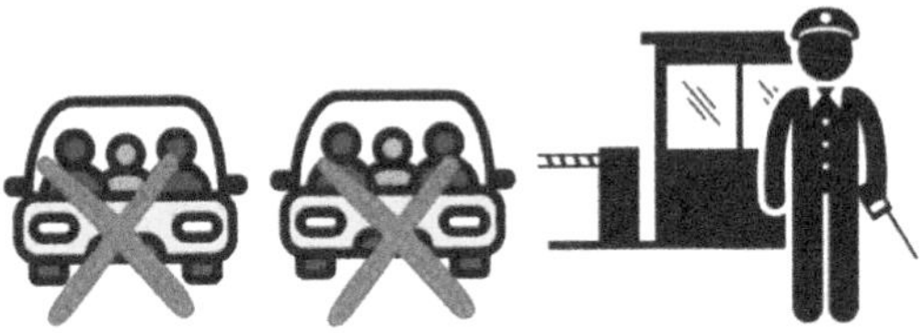

The system runs low on Good Guys so no longer able to function properly.

Topic 1: Problem Created

What We Don't See

By assuming my hypothesis was true, my health improved. Here is my more science-y educated guess of what I think is going on that we cannot see. With no amazing microscope, but with many Kahn Academy videos, I decided to focus in on the lymphatic system. Very roughly explained, our lymph nodes are supposed to scan the passing interstellar fluid in search of harmful pathogens. It then grabs them up to do what they are meant to do. Thus, creating the necessary Attackers to fight the Bad Guys it is grabbing up. If, during the scanning process, the items seen are not harmful, they are left alone and drift their way to the surface of our skin.

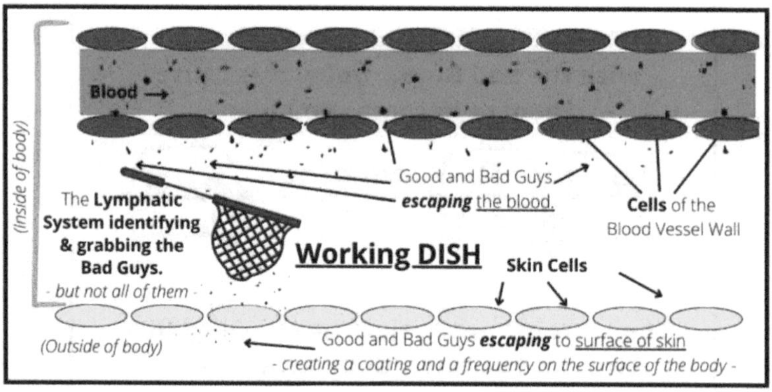

Keep in mind, not all Bad Guys nor all Good Guys leak their way out of the blood vessels. Only a small percentage do. The rest continue to their destinations. This small percentage, though, is all that is needed. The skin is the equal sign with the same frequency on both sides, inside and outside of the body. This matching frequency allows the Good Guys to have an exit road. It allows them to avoid being grouped with the Bad Guys. It allows DISH to do its second job.

If, for some reason, there is too much fluid and the exit route is hampered, these Good Guys end up hanging out too long in Excess Lymph Land. The lymph nodes end up grabbing them up and pushing them through the system with the Bad Guy. When this occurs, if they are grouped with a Bad Guy, they now become an enemy.

When I took supplements, I needed to make sure my body was sorting. Some of the supplements needed to be able to come to the surface of the skin otherwise it could become part of the problem. I think holding these supplements worked better than just taking them. It was all

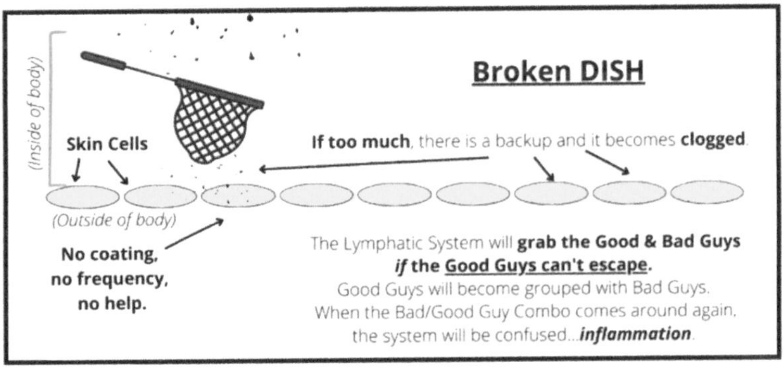

about creating the frequency coating on the surface of the skin—they needed exit ramps. With this coating and the body keeping the Good Guys it needed, sometimes the supplements weren't even needed to be taken. The sorting prevented the body from rejecting the Good Guys. Thus, stopping the loss automatically forced the replenishing of the depleted supply. Without the coating—automatic or manual—the risk was there of the Good Guy becoming grouped with a Bad Guy. Something the body would start rejecting. This rejecting down the road, if the information is not reprogrammed, I believe will result in inflammation.

Allow me to repeat this one more time. This is a HUGE factor.

If the sorting system is NOT working,

taking supplements to remedy the problem

becomes part of the problem.

This was where I was stuck until I realized if I held the supplements for ten minutes before or twenty minutes after, it was enough to prevent this from happening. I manually did the work of creating this coating so I could take the supplements without them becoming a part of the problem. If it was a supplement I needed to take throughout the day, I just ended up holding it continuously.

How Bad Guys Build Up in the Body

Looking deeper, I learned Bad Guys could build up on an organ or a meridian. Meridians are closely related to the organs they are named after. I believe the building up of these Bad Guys is related to the meridian clock. Allow me to explain.

The body follows a meridian clock. It basically is a fixed pattern corresponding to time on a clock. It consists of twelve two-hour segments. The body follows this pattern to *work through* each meridian on a daily basis. Depending on what time of the day my DISH malfunctioned, the group of Bad

Guys would have the potential to become attached to the meridian and its corresponding organs. If my body was able to neutralize it before the two-hour window was over, it would not get stuck. If the body couldn't neutralize it, the Bad Guy would get carried over to the next meridian.

Some meridians may be weaker and/or have more problems than other ones. And as I proceeded throughout my day, different Bad Guys would come into contact with my body. If my shield was up, nothing. If my shield was down, add it to the pile.

Back to the road analogy: the pothole gets bigger (Bad Guy buildup) if there is any damage already there. It is just like potholes in a road. If there is no damage, the road is barely affected by the traffic.

When I realized what was going on here during this process, I became really discouraged at the idea of how long this was going to take. But what else was I to do if this was the only way I could regain my health?

Meridian Clock Guide

5-7 am: Large Intestines
7-9 am: Stomach
9-11 am: Spleen
11-1 pm: Heart
1-3 pm: Small Intestines
3-5 pm: Bladder
5-7 pm: Kidney
7-9 pm: Pericardium (Heart Constrictor)
9-11 pm: Triple Warmer (Immune system)
11-1 am: Gall Bladder
1-3 am: Liver
3-5 am: Lung

When It Gets Tricky

Enter nutrition and hormones. I am sure you have heard the saying that circulates around about how we need to let food be our medicine. I agreed with this statement. But this statement was not helping me. What I needed to eat I was unable to eat. I was acquiring new food and environmental allergies daily, or so it seemed. Why was that?

Nutrients and hormones are our Helpers. How do they turn on us?

It took me almost seven years to figure it out. But I now know this is what was happening to me.

1. Body Fighting Bad Guy

Remember, nothing can be created or destroyed. The Bad Guy needed to become something else when it was conquered. It became Byproduct. The body now needed to deal with the Bad Guy and its Byproduct, two separate problems. (Or technically three if I add in the combination of Bad Guy and Byproduct together.) The job just became bigger. If this bigger job becomes too big, our body's immune system is at risk of flipping the switch. Why? Too many cars.

Not only is this occurring, but our organs are creating extra *sweat* from working harder. (Even more traffic.)

2. Danger Zone

Let's say we are taking in the Good Guy we need to fight the Bad Guy. These Good Guys are winning. They are converting these Bad Guys into Byproduct. However, the current Good Guys are not the ones designed to fight the Byproduct. The Byproduct is the Bad Guy changed, so of course this could easily be the case. At this point, if we don't call in a new type of Good Guy for reinforcement to fight the Byproduct, this Byproduct could build up. If the original Good Guys continue to attack the Bad Guy, excessive amounts of Byproduct will hurt the system. The system will slow down because it doesn't have what it needed to fight both. (Traffic jam likely.)

Putting in more water doesn't always unclog the sink.

---

3. The Mixing Point

With all of this extra *traffic*, like my coffee filter experience, the Good Guy roads may become blocked. The Good Guys, who were targeting the Bad Guys and making progress, may become grouped with those same Bad Guys. When this happens, the Good Guys' level drops in two ways.

- Being used up from doing a big job of fighting Bad Guys.
- Being rejected with the Bad Guy because they can't escape Lymph Land before getting grabbed up and grouped with them.

Adding more of the same Good Guys at this point to focus on the original Bad Guy alone will only make the problem worse. However, there are two things that would help at this point.

- Hold the Good Guys so they have an exit ramp.
- Hold and take the Good Guys needed to fight the Byproduct.

This Mixing Point is where I believe the switch gets flipped. The tug-of-war begins. The body does and doesn't want to fight. It tries to slow down the loss of Good Guys. This slowing down may happen with inflammation, candida flare-up, thyroid slowing down, or other methods associated with having a weak immune system.

Topic 2: The Vicious Cycle

Looking at the problem backwards again from the way I figured it out, when Job Two (Sorting) failed, it caused Job One (Protecting) to malfunction because the body was failing to hold onto the nutrients it needed to detox and function properly.

Things became jumbled when Job Two malfunctioned.

While the sorting system was working, the body was able to easily identify Good from Bad. It could even see more than one Bad Guy at a time. As long as the organs were strong and the sorting continued, the body could handle it. But when the load became too much for the lymph roads, misinformation began. With this misinformation, the body started to run low on the nutrients it needed to function properly. When this happened, it became even easier to receive the unwanted misinformation. They fed off of each other in a vicious cycle. A cycle that needed to be corrected. But how? It does not matter what flipped it. The problem was that it was flipped. Having been flipped, there was a compromised system trying to do its job still. Flipping the switch back would stop the problem. It would get us back to the side of before *something happened.*

As I mentioned earlier, there are three players at work when this switch is flipped. We have the Good Guys, the Bad Guys, and the Byproduct. In order to fix the flipped switch, flip it back. This is easier said than done because of how the Good Guys and Bad Guys may have interacted with each other. Unmixing some things is easier than unmixing others.

Plus, if the misinformation happened too long before being caught, missing information may have started to occur. Depending on the type of Good Guys missing, the missing information in the body could literally make the body forget what it was supposed to be doing. It lost its programming software. It needed to be re-plugged in and rebooted. The organs either forgot what they were supposed to do or were no longer receiving the signal. Insane, right?

I do recall at one point my leg didn't receive the message my brain sent it to take a step forward. I was walking across the kitchen floor when my right foot failed to realize it was its turn again. It didn't move. I fell flat to the ground. I was so glad I wasn't holding my baby at the time!

Could it be possible for the detox organs to be in the same situation? My lab tests said my organs were working properly. Were they not getting the signal? It sure felt like the body was missing information.

Because the brain was not getting the nutrients it needed, maybe other organs stopped receiving all the information they needed to do their jobs as well. This resulted in more misinformation; thus, the vicious cycle continued.

The best way to prevent needing to reprogram It

is to prevent the errant programming

from happening in the first place.

Chain Reaction

Mis-Information causes essential nutrients or hormones to be rejected.

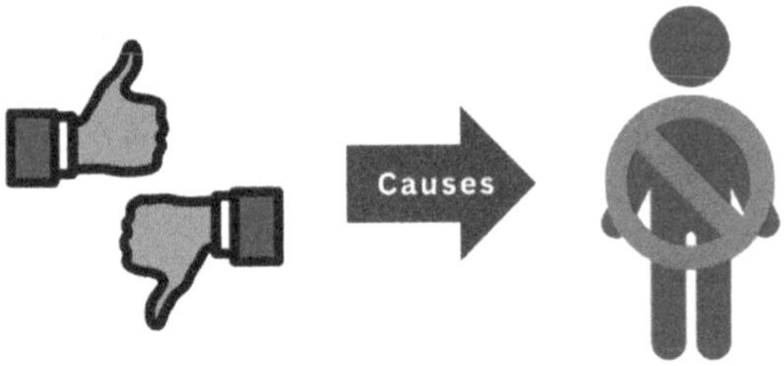

This rejection causes a deficiency.

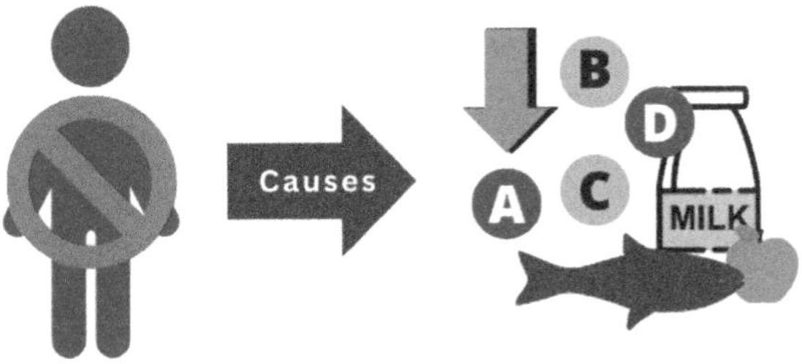

The deficiency causes missing information.

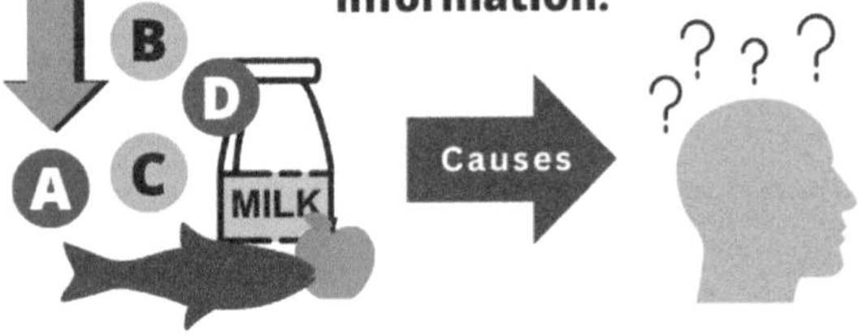

Missing information prevents body from functioning properly.

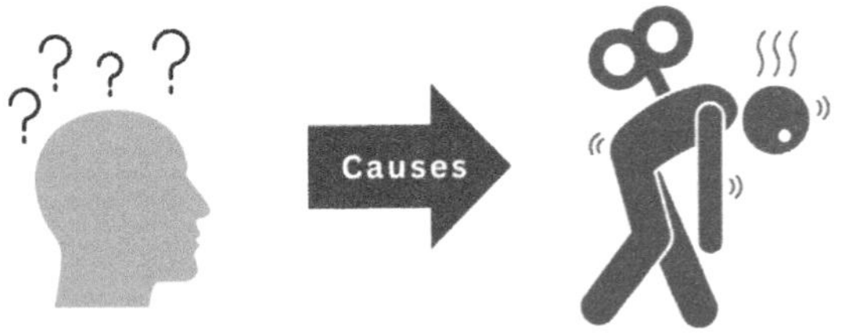

(As well as lack of nutrients for other organs.)

Topic 3: Problem Avoided

Because of how misinformation and missing information feed off of each other in a vicious cycle, it is best to avoid the problem altogether. For those with a working DISH, they may just need to keep up with the Big Five. For others, if they are like me, they can't rely on the Big Five Assumptions being enough. I needed to be proactive during times of potentially reaching the saturation point. I needed to be mindful of when Excess Lymph Land was getting crowded and avoid the buildup in order to avoid the cycle from beginning in the first place.

How to Be Proactive

There were two primary ways of being proactive during potential times of inflammation or other illnesses or treatments.

My Environment

- Anything I ate or drank, I kept in my energy field for thirty minutes.
- Any medication I took for fighting the Bad Guy or the problem he caused, I kept in my energy field continually until the Bad Guy was gone (days/months).
- Be aware of my environment.
- Avoid energy fields stronger than mine.

My Battle

- Determine what part of the body was being affected/targeted.
- For example, intestines, lungs, bones.

- Research what Good Guys those body parts needed. Major or minor Good Guys, full list would be ideal.
- Keep those Good Guys in my energy field at all times to keep an exit ramp available. Usually ranging from full contact to in the same room.

What This Looks Like

During my health journey, I had hit bumps in the road. But I think understanding DISH helped me to get through it. According to my calculations and patterns I had been observing, I had *released* plastic from my body. I knew I was heading for a train wreck, though, because I could not figure out what to hold to help with the Byproduct of plastic. True to form, forty-eight hours after the release of plastic, when the Byproduct kicked in, my stomach pain began. I'm not saying I'm a tough cookie, but when stomach pain is so common that going to the hospital doesn't even cross my mind... I delayed two days before going in only to find out my appendix was ruptured! The CAT scan said it had ruptured two days earlier!

There was noticeable infection, the procedure took longer than expected, and I was in my 50s and overweight (plastic does a number on the liver, but that is for a different book). These were all strong potential candidates for readmission after being released from the hospital. The doctors even said they had noticed that for some reason if a patient stayed until day five, readmission was lowest. I was dismissed the third day. I was told I had a fifty/fifty chance of being readmitted.

But I think Altering Fields to Enable Recovery (AFTER) helped me. This is how I did it. Before my CAT scan, I needed to drink some liquid. I made sure I knew what the liquid was for information later. (Being aware of my surroundings protocol for AFTER at work here.) It was potassium iodine. I felt like my DISH was working during the CAT scan, so there was a plus sign. Before the surgery, I sprinkled on the top of my head the supplements I had been holding. After surgery, I left the TV off. When I was given my medication, I didn't want to be asked what I was doing, so when the nurse's back was turned, I would lick the pill and rub it on my forearm to have it on the outside. I would then take it. I would hold the IV tube on my core as often as possible to have the antibiotics be on the outside and the inside.

When it was time to go home (and this was during COVID, so no visitors), I asked if I could take my IV and the empty drip bag home with me to show my kids what saved their mom. They agreed. So thankful! I needed to hold this bag in and out of my energy field many times those first few days. On day five, I needed to hold it continuously for about five hours. It was during the toughest time. I have no doubt in my mind if I wasn't doing AFTER, I would have been readmitted to the hospital at this time. But alas, there is no way to prove or disprove that.

I continued to do AFTER during my recovery. For example, I was very glad I knew what I drank for the CAT scan. I needed to hold onto potassium iodine for several days while my body was removing the radiation from the CAT scan. Did it work? Well, when I went in for my post-surgery checkup, they were surprised at how well I was doing and how few issues I had. I attribute this to AFTER. (BTW: this was not my first surgery.)

Personal Examples

For me, it was sunflower seeds. Sunflower seeds (not a common allergen) are high in panthodic acid (vitamin B5). When I ate sunflower seeds, my body saw this as reinforcements to fight the virus attacking my nervous system. Fighting the virus caused inflammation. This inflammation caused the panthodic acid to become grouped with the virus. As a result, whenever I ate sunflower seeds, I fought the virus. But they are grouped... I also fought (rejected) panthodic acid. The rear guards didn't want to run out of the panthodic acid. The body powered down and allowed the virus to stay. The lesser of the two evils was letting the virus stay. The body can't run on empty. I could not get rid of the virus. It was either both or neither. Tug-of-war (chronic inflammation).

My body could not do neither. The allergic reaction to the sunflower seeds was because when I ate them, my body saw this as an opportunity to fight the virus. But fight it, I should not. Nor could I safely do it because it wasn't enough of what my body needed to win the fight. There wasn't enough panthodic acid in the sunflower seeds to do the job completely (or in my case panthodic acid and oxytocin).

I saw this pattern happening repeatedly. The organ causing me woes needed the nutrients that my body was deficient in. My body was allergic to the foods containing those nutrients. The foods with those nutrients in them were enough to give the body the incentive to rebel, but they were not strong enough to win the battle. These Good Guys were being mixed with the Bad Guys. This caused the Good Guys to be misidentified. ***The switch was flipped.***

I know there are malabsorption challenges. I also know sometimes the body is unable to use the nutrient at all. I also know sometimes a nutrient is removed when removing something harmful from the body. But maybe a fourth thing is a factor as well. Maybe the nutrient is just flat out being rejected. The body saw the Good Guy as being on the wrong team.

Thought to Ponder

Would the Mixing Point that occurs when factoring DISH explain this?

- Have you or do you know someone who developed a food allergy after an illness?
- Is it possible the Good Guy in this food became joined with the Bad Guy or its Byproduct from this illness?
- Let's take a look at what the Centers for Disease Control (CDC) has to say about chronic fatigue syndrome (CFS)—also called myalgic encephalomyelitis (ME)—while keeping the DISH Mixing Point in mind.
- People with ME/CFS often have their illness begin in a way that reminds them of getting the flu. This has made researchers suspect an infection may trigger ME/CFS. In addition, about one in ten people who become infected with Epstein-Barr virus, Ross River virus, or

Coxiella burnetti will develop a set of symptoms that meet the criteria for ME/CFS.[47]

- Is the virus the **something happened** that caused the switch to be flipped?
- Did the saturation point occur causing the mixing of Good Guys with Bad Guys and the resulting chronic inflammation is the body having a tug-of-war battle of trying to hold onto these Good Guys?
- Is the reason it is so hard to pin down the problem because the trigger could be anything?
- Should we stop looking for so many triggers and instead look at what the trigger did?

The CDC website also says, "It is possible that ME/CFS is caused by a change in the person's immune system and the way it responds to infection or stress."[48]

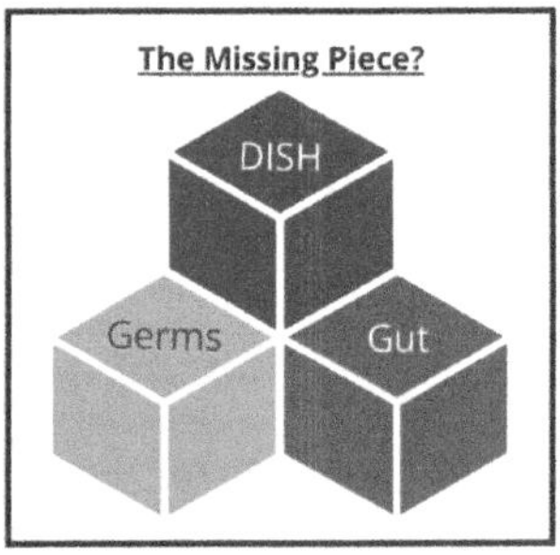

---

[47] Centers for Disease Control. "Myalgic Encephalomyelitis / Chronic Fatigue Syndrome Possible Causes- Infections." Centers for Disease Control and Prevention. Last reviewed 12 July 2018. https://www.cdc.gov/me-cfs/about/possible-causes.html.

[48] Centers for Disease Control. "Myalgic Encephalomyelitis / Chronic Fatigue Syndrome Possible Causes- Immune System Changes." Centers for Disease Control and Prevention. Last reviewed 12 July 2018. https://www.cdc.gov/me-cfs/about/possible-causes.html.

- Is this revealing the flipped switch?
- Is the fact this switch has been flipped what really matters?

Scientists have mentioned there is a connection between the immune system and the lymphatic system. Maybe this DISH is just an expansion on this idea. Maybe understanding DISH would help us to better understand the relationship between these two systems. Maybe it is the missing piece for connecting the two parts of good health: fight germs and healthy gut. I know the better I understood DISH, the more my health improved.

Conclusion for Chapter 5

If we accept the simple basis that the body's job is to be well, and it wants to be well, the perspective changes. If the body is attacking itself, either it has alienated itself from its primary objective, or it sees this attacking as the lesser of the two evils.

Predisposition for the Trigger Being Flipped

We are told there are seven factors that impact immune tolerance.

1. **My Sex**—seventy-eight percent are females.
2. **Genetics**—Certain disorders run in families.
3. **Having an Autoimmune Disease**.
    - Twenty-five percent of patients have three or more.
    - To me, this is circular reasoning. How did the first one get there?

4. Obesity

- Seventy-two percent of the population is overweight in the United States.
- Is the obesity causing it or a result of it, though?

5. Smoking and Exposure to Toxic Agents—Not only do these toxins alter gene expression but maybe they also make too many Bad Guys present. (Traffic Jam in Excess Lymph Land.)

6. Certain Medications—Are we adding more Guys to an already crowded system without giving the Helpers (Good Guys) a way out?

7. Infections—Is this the **something happened** factor?

Looking at this list was frustrating to me. I had no control over the first two. The third one was me; I was not looking forward to getting more. Four through seven were not me. Why was I still given the problem? I felt so helpless.

What if there was only one thing determining immune tolerance? A working DISH.

If I look back over the list, I see a bunch of Bad Guys. Maybe even enough Bad Guys to clog the system and cause a switch to be flipped. What if knowing DISH is there and being mindful of the Mixing Point potentially happening during an illness or toxin exposure is a way to avoid the switch being flipped? Would it help make recovery easier or prevent the immune system from receiving misinformation, which in turn would start the vicious cycle that just might be ME/CFS?

Could I take back control of my health by resetting this switch?

In order to understand how to even do that, I needed to understand these Bad Guys.

CHAPTER 6: CRASH COURSE ON BAD GUY BEHAVIOR

Understanding what we are up against.

Opening Story: Lying on the Floor with Jars

When going through a rough patch in life, the tiny little grains of hope sprinkled throughout are so powerful. In motivational speaker circles the story of the drowning mice is usually circulated. If you haven't heard of it before, it was an experiment done in 1957. They would put mice in tubes of water to see how long they would survive. They averaged about fifteen minutes. They also noticed they were able to extend this time to almost sixty hours just by giving these mice hope. [49] Hope that it would not always be this way. Like those mice, I found some hope to cling to.

During this time for me, I had camped out in a spot in front of my wood stove in the living room. The power was cut to this part of the house. I was wearing my pajamas still. I'm not sure if I even took them off for over a month. They were safe. They were made out of cotton. They had a drawstring for the waist. No metal zippers or buttons. The pull-on top was the same. In front of me was my desperate attempt to find the frequency that would bring me back to normal. Two

[49] Richter, Dr. Curt P. "The Power of Hope—Curt P. Richter's 'Hope Experiment.'" E-motivation.net. Last accessed 27 March 2023. https://www.e-motivation.net/the-power-of-hope-curt-p-richters-hope-experiment/.

laundry baskets filled with jars of many sizes. Jars filled with water and combinations of homeopathic remedies. I was starting to feel fatigued and dizzy again. I again grabbed half a dozen jars and pulled them close to me as I lay down on the aged carpet. It worked until it didn't. Again.

I rolled away from them and looked out the window toward the sky. Early spring. Too cold still to be outside, but the sunshine was nice. I sighed. I felt the need for the jars again. I rolled back over and just grabbed one. It worked. Until it didn't. Pause, think. Something was going on here. Rotating these jars in and out of my immediate surroundings was doing something. This was the beginning of realizing the patterns taking place before my eyes. It took me over two years of seeing these patterns before I had the *aha* experience I mentioned in the previous chapter. Before I realized it, I was manually changing my DISH frequency since it would not do it independently.

What I was manually doing to create this artificial DISH was working. I think it would suffice to say this was what the body automatically did when the DISH did work. I just needed to copy it until I figured out why my DISH didn't. This didn't happen until years later when I realized how I was losing my Good Guys. The information I have shared with you.

Overview

If you could picture a schoolyard bully, the first thing you would want to do is to just not be picked on. You would hope the bully would just leave you alone. Fly under the radar. But as time went by, I became stronger—whether that be mentally or physically. Now, if I saw a bully picking on someone else, I may decide to intervene. This was kind of what the two main levels of dealing with Bad Guys looked like.

The first level is just what I call maintaining mode: holding what I needed to hold so my DISH could do its jobs. Doing this, I was able to function normally. I was doing this most of the time.

The second level is proactive mode: leveling up to remove the problem the body was unable to fight in maintaining mode. This required doing a batch. Doing a batch was time consuming, hard on the body, scary uncharted territory, and liberating. It was always followed by a jump of improvement in my health.

But before I could level up to this proactive mode, I needed to study the Bad Guys and understand their behavior. In this chapter I will share what my reconnaissance mission revealed. It will conclude the first half of this book. This chapter is like learning the grammar parts of a sentence. The next successive chapters will be about making them into actual sentences. So don't feel intimidated by this chapter. It will make more sense once it is combined with the rest of the book.

To beat my enemy, know my enemy.

Topic 1: DISH Vocabulary

Terminology

Like any field of study, to really understand it we need to understand the vocabulary of it. Since I was in uncharted territory, I created my own vocabulary for this new concept. I have tried to simplify the concept as best I could. It may sound complicated. I didn't make it up. I didn't make the rules. I just observed and noticed these patterns over the past decade and gave names to the patterns and their contributing parts.

Borrowed Words from Acupuncture

I am not an acupuncturist, nor do I feel like I have even scraped the tip of the iceberg on the details of how to use acupuncture as a treatment. However, I do believe these meridians and acupuncture points affected my health. I needed to be aware of the main meridian locations on my body. I also needed to use the meridian clock to narrow down my problem areas. These will become major factors as I work through the *batches* I refer to later.

As a refresher from page one hundred twelve, a meridian clock is the twenty-four-hour period of time split into twelve two-hour windows. Each one of those windows has a meridian and organs corresponding to it. It is when the body targets the given meridian and the organs corresponding to it. Yes, there is also a governing vessel (roughly translated, my skeletal system) and a conception vessel (having to do with reproduction) and the *qi* meridian. I'll admit the *qi* meridian is still a total mystery to me. I'm not sure where it fits in. An easy way to look at these acupuncture points, meridians, and organs is like a highway system. The meridians are the roads that lead to the organs (city). The acupuncture points are the traffic lights on the way from point A to point B on those roads. I needed to be aware of these roads, traffic lights, and the schedule they kept.

Unique DISH Vocabulary Words

Words can have different meanings for different people. I chose a fresh set of new words to better explain what I figured out. I have tried to group them together to help make it easier to learn.

First, we have the Players.

1. **Bad Guy:** Anything in the body that shouldn't be there. The normal word used for this (toxins) means different things to different people, so I prefer to use a unique word.
2. **Target:** This is the Bad Guy being focused on.
3. **Gatekeeper:** Another word I use for target when holding it enabled me to work on everything else under it in the batch. Picture a triangle. The Gatekeeper is at the top of the triangle.
4. **Byproduct:** What is left when a Bad Guy is destroyed.
5. **POOP:** Product of Other Product. This is the Byproduct of the Byproduct. Sometimes it was so harmful to my body that I needed to treat it as a Bad Guy as well.
6. **Kingpin:** This is a significant target grouping several Bad Guys together.
7. **Mimicker:** A Bad Guy that is mimicking an essential nutrient or hormone (Good Guy) the body needs.
8. **Good Guy:** What the body needs to function properly. This could be a vitamin, mineral, good bacteria, hormone, etc.

Second, we have where these Players are located.

1. Pillars: This is the name I gave the areas the body consisted of. It refers to the twelve meridians, the governing vessel, the conception vessel, the *qi* meridian, the nervous system, and corresponding groups of organs. Not all pillars are involved every time.

2. Batches: This is a group of Bad Guys with or without Good Guys in tow. These batches can be formed in three different ways. By knowing how they are formed it is easier to be able to fix the problem.

a. **Exposure:** I was exposed to the items at the same time.

✓ For example: Styrofoam and coffee.

b. **Resemblance:** The items were like each other.

✓ For example: kerosene and gasoline.

c. **Proximity:** The items were in the same location.

✓ For example: collagen and rheumatoid arthritis (bones).

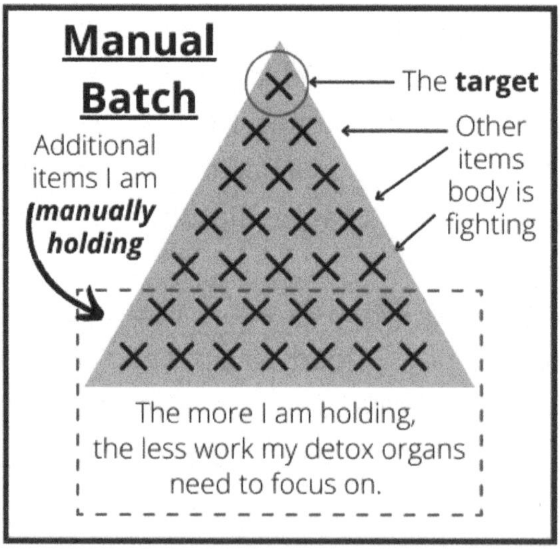

Thirdly, we have what is happening to the Players. Each Player will go through four steps.

1. **Identify:** This is when the Bad Guy first appears on the scene. I needed my body to recognize what it was.
2. **Neutralize:** This is when an individual Bad Guy* has been singled out from the rest of the Bad Guys in the batch. The body has targeted it to where it will become strong enough to now fight the particular Bad Guy on a solitary level.
3. **Release:** This is when the Bad Guy is on top of all the pillars—the entire body involved. Once this happens, the body is able to neutralize this individual Bad Guy everywhere the body is being affected by it. The individual Bad Guy becomes a nonissue for the body.
4. **Remove:** This released individual Bad Guy is now just hanging out and waiting for the Bad Guys it is connected to to also be released. Once it and its comrades are all released, they can then be safely removed from the body.

*Or *a stuck group* (homogeneous batch)—this will make sense later. I just didn't want to be contradictory and cause confusion when I bring this point up later.

Lastly, we have a few other terminology words I use.

1. **Hold or holding:** This is just having the Bad Guy within my energy field. The distance can vary from skin contact on a specific spot to being a few inches from my body (usually).
2. **DISH is a shield:** I use these two words interchangeably. Remember, the S in DISH stands for shield. These words are referring to the energy field around my

body. The status of the shield determines whether or not DISH is doing its two jobs.

3. Shields up: My DISH is working properly by protecting the body with a tiny little force field. This shield is giving off a frequency. DISH is doing its two jobs.

- Protecting
- Sorting

4. Shields down: My DISH is failing to do its two jobs of protecting and sorting.

5. Batch neutralizing session: This is when I sit and slowly introduce into my energy field parts of my environment, essential oils, remedies, food, supplements, and anything else associated with the batch.

6. Retraining the body: The process of correcting missing or misinformation.

Hold or Holding

- Having an object in my immediate energy field.
- The energy field size varies from 1 in. to 6 ft., depending on the person
- It may or may not be in physical contact to my person.

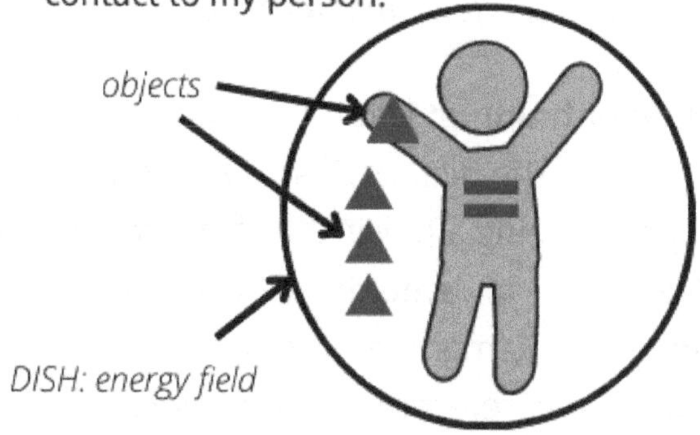

Topic 2: Four Concepts to Understand

This next section is important. It will explain the four vocabulary words that missed the lineup. They warranted being elaborated on. They are the moving parts of what is happening. They mesh together so much, sometimes it is difficult to see where one begins and the other ends. Understanding them, though, made it possible to find the target I was looking for when I chose to start manually making my DISH.

1. Triggers

When I have a reaction to something, is it because my body saw this as an opportunity to remove a Bad Guy from my system? I see this triggering of an allergy different than the norm. I'm looking at it sort of backwards, I guess. Instead of looking at the problem that created it, maybe it's what the allergen started.

Two possible scenarios.

➢ If a Bad Guy is in the body and the body is exposed to the same Bad Guy, it sees it as an opportunity to leave without the body having to process it out. (Because technically it is still processing it out if we accept the concept of DISH, but the detox organs just aren't the ones required to do the work.)

- This causes problems if it is tied to another Bad Guy.
- This also causes problems if it tries to take Good Guys with it.

➢ If what would normally be considered a Good Guy is introduced into the system, the body may see these reinforcements as an opportunity to remove the Bad Guy. But if it doesn't have enough Good Guys to do the job, the body reacts to it.

For example, in order for me to remove my food allergy of egg, I needed to take supplements of omega, vitamin D, and zinc with it, as well as hold them. I would also only trigger it once a day by eating egg. It gave my body time to process out whatever it needed to without trying to do too much at once. Hypothetically, because vaccinations used to be grown only on egg, I received tuberculosis (TB) with egg. My sorting didn't work, so it stayed combined. Now, whenever I ate egg, my body saw it as an opportunity to get rid of TB/egg. But it couldn't. It still wasn't sorting correctly to be able to remove just TB.

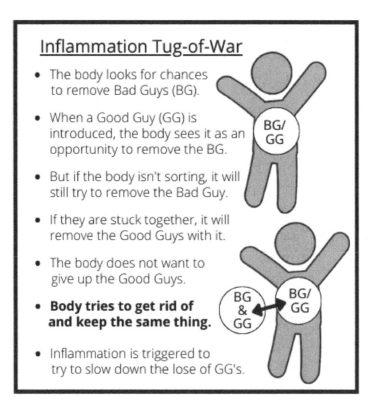

Inflammation Tug-of-War

- The body looks for chances to remove Bad Guys (BG).
- When a Good Guy (GG) is introduced, the body sees it as an opportunity to remove the BG.
- But if the body isn't sorting, it will still try to remove the Bad Guy.
- If they are stuck together, it will remove the Good Guys with it.
- The body does not want to give up the Good Guys.
- **Body tries to get rid of and keep the same thing.**
- Inflammation is triggered to try to slow down the lose of GG's.

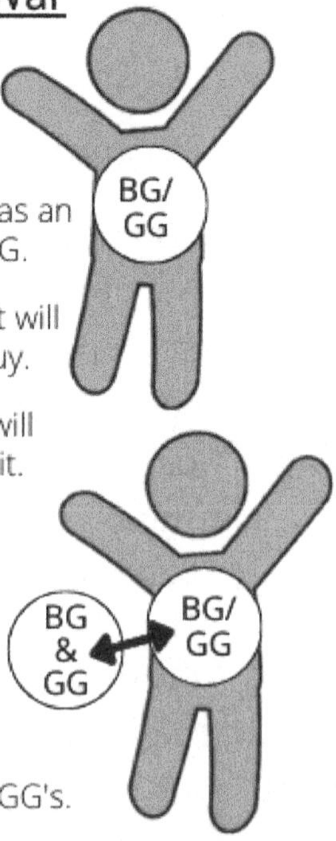

2. Frenemies

Nothing can be created or destroyed. Destroying the Bad Guy creates Bad Guy corpses—Byproduct. They need to be dealt with also. Focusing on managing the Byproduct was the way to keep the body fighting the Bad Guy. To keep hauling the dead Bad Guys away so they don't become tied to the Good Guys doing their job.

- ***Mixing Point Reached***

What helped me will hurt me. By the Good Guys doing their job well there will be a battle (inflammation). This battle may cause a chain reaction as mentioned previously. So, what I needed in order to fight the problem would also become a part of the problem unless, of course, it had an exit ramp to avoid being combined with the Bad Guy. The exit ramp is automatic for some people, but not for me.

The type of frenemy I was dealing with would depend on the type of batch it was. This is so extensive it will be covered more in Chapters 7 and 8.

- ***Harmful Byproduct***

Sometimes the Byproduct (dead Bad Guys) was more harmful than the Bad Guys. One example is if a person is infected with the loa loa parasite. The toxins these parasites give off when dying—if the infestation is high—can cause people to fall into a coma. Therefore, the standard parasite treatment cannot be implemented.[50]

---

[50] Centers for Disease Control and Prevention. "Parasites—Loiasis: Treatment." Centers for Disease Control and Prevention. Last reviewed 20 January 2015. https://www.cdc.gov/parasites/loiasis/treatment.html.

Another example is the Byproduct of plastic. When poisoned with plastic, removing it caused more damage to the body than allowing it to just stay there.[51]

3. Pathway

The Bad Guy always followed a pattern as it worked its way through a batch. Recognizing this pathway enabled me to notice what was coming and what to research. It also enabled me to see progress. Progress I wouldn't have recognized if I didn't realize what was going on. It also later helped me in recognizing the cycling that was happening. (Cycling is the next term I'll cover.)

Each Bad Guy needed to be confronted when it was on the top of the pillar. Allow me to explain with a game analogy.

COLORS GAME ANALOGY

I've seen them advertised on my iPhone, so I'm hoping you have too. The game consists of a collection of glasses or tubes or some similar type of clear container. Inside of these containers you will see a liquid or balls or sand or a similar type of item with a variety of colors mixed together. The object of the game is to move the objects around until all of the objects with the same color are in the same tube. This is where my analogy becomes different. However, if you can

[51] Division of Toxicology and Environmental Medicine. "Public Health Statement; Vinyl Chloride CAS#: 75-01-4." Department of Health and Human Services. July 2006. https://www.atsdr.cdc.gov/ToxProfiles/tp20-c1-b.pdf.

picture this game in your head, I would like to use it to clarify what happens.

A. Bad Guy reveals itself: This would be when I would need a new homeopathic remedy. In this analogy, it would be the color being on top of one tube, but the same color would be present in different layers throughout the tube as well.

B. Bad Guy is ready to be neutralized: This is when I would make a batch with this Bad Guy being the target. In this analogy, the one color I was targeting would be merged to the top of a tube. It is no longer dispersed throughout the given tube. The way it surfaces to the top is by having everything above it be neutral, whether by the body doing its job or holding those items in my energy field.

C. Bad Guy is ready to be released: This is when the Bad Guy I am targeting is showing up everywhere as the problem in my body. In this analogy, all of the tubes have the same color on top. Some of them may have the color throughout their tube as well during this stage.

D. Two things happen during the release: In the beginning this required holding many objects (usually a dozen or more). But the more I neutralized what was in the way, the faster this process would go.

- *The body is now strong enough to fight this Bad Guy.* In this analogy, it is allowed to dump the first layer off of the tubes only when all tubes have the same color on the top. This color is now a nonissue in the body, by itself. But it now needs to be released from the other colors associated with it.
- *The Bad Guy starts to be removed from the body.* In this analogy, if the color is nowhere else in the tube, the color has been removed from this tube only. If it is still elsewhere in the tube,

the colors that are above it and preventing it from coming to the surface need to be neutralized. Once everything above it is neutralized, it will be sent to the top to meet up with the same color. When that occurs, it, too, can now be dumped and removed from the body.

E. Bad Guy is Removed: Once the color is completely gone in all tubes, then it is removed. FYI: It took almost six years for egg to complete this process. However, I reiterate, I was still figuring it out. I don't know if it could have gone faster if I understood sooner what was going on.

4. Cycling

This is not something I deliberately did, but it is something the body did on its own. If I failed to realize this is what was going on, it usually made it more difficult to narrow down the problem.

This usually happened if the target was missing. When muscle testing for the source of the problem, it will keep changing in its results—meaning minute by minute if not second by second changes. Some attribute this to muscle testing being inaccurate. The results keep changing. Actually, no. The target—probably a Kingpin—was just missing.

For example, when I was at my nutritionist, he noticed that 1, 2, 3, 4, 5, & 6 were a problem for me. But when he started working on how to fix them, only 4 & 6 were showing up as the problem. And before he even went down the road of focusing on them, they were no longer the problem, but 1 & 2 were. My body was actually working on 1–6, but it could only do a few at a time before it would break to the next one (or group) because the *top item* was missing. When the top item, #7, was found, it enabled me to work automatically on batching 1–6 in all combinations without needing them. I only needed #7—the top X (target) in the Growing a Batch infographic (elaborated on in future chapters).

If a Bad Guy disappeared and reappeared again, it was frustrating. Was it working or not? Yes and no—it depended. This was where it started to get complicated because of the need to pull so much knowledge together. This is when pattern watching paid off. But in order to pattern watch, I needed to be aware of the meridian clock. I needed to have been taking notes. I needed to be searching for repeats and how often they occurred.

- ***Good Cycling: Two signs of progress forward.***
    - Same batch on different meridian clock time segments.
    - Same batch plus more items on the strongest or same meridian clock segment.
- ***Bad Cycling: Signs of no progress being made.***
    - Same batch on same meridian clock forty-eight hours later.
    - Something is missing.
        - Am I needing to hold more or different Good Guys?
        - Am I trying to do too many Bad Guys at once?
    - Not strong enough.
        - Is it possible to break the Bad Guy down into even smaller pieces?

        - Is there a stronger energy field preventing me from making progress?
        - Am I exposing myself to an allergen?
        - Am I lacking the needed Good Guy to win this battle?

- ***Neutral Cycling: Neither good nor bad, just is.***
    - Slow progress.
        - Need to hold many things.
        - Sporadic—no visible pattern.
    - Missing a Gatekeeper or Kingpin.

Topic 3: Five Basic Principles

The pile of information is continuing to build up, so you can probably see what I mean by the idea of it being a simple concept but difficult to implement. We are now going to take the players, the places, and the concepts we know so far and dump them all into five basic principles. I have called this process of implementing all this information Altering Fields to Enable Recovery (AFTER). Doing this is what enabled me to get out of maintaining mode and into proactive mode. Proactive mode was the process of digging deeper to find what caused the problem in the first place, so I could flip the switch back.

1. Batches

What a Batch Looks Like

The easiest way for me to visualize batches was to look at them as triangles. The top of the triangle is the target. Everything else is related to it. However, triangles overlap with each other. I wanted to target the smaller triangles before tackling the larger triangles. Working on one item in a

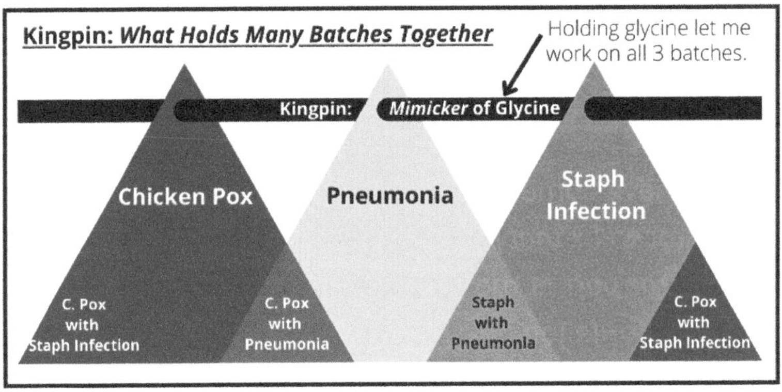

triangle may be related to an item in a different triangle. A rod would connect these triangles to each other. This rod is a Kingpin. It would be a Mimicker of something the body needed. It would be the main target of different batches.

How a Batch Is Described

The better I understood batches, the easier it was to maneuver the Bad Guy I was targeting into the top position where I needed him to be. I will be dedicating the next three chapters to batches. For now, just know there are three ways to describe a batch: how it's formed, its status, and how it's grouped.

A. How it's formed
- Exposure
- Proximity
- Resemblance

B. Its status
- Complete
- Incomplete
- Canceled

C. How it's grouped
- Heterogeneous
- Homogeneous
- Mimicker

2. Strongest to Weakest

When we have something wrong with ourselves, we go and ask a doctor to fix *that part*. Well, welcome to opposite world. Let's say *that part* is the weak pillar. *That part* is not strong enough to do *its* job. That is why *it* is broken. Something I discovered is I needed to focus on the strongest pillar first, not the weakest. I didn't need to have the weak pillar push itself up; I needed to use a stronger pillar to pull it up. I needed to let the stronger pillar do the heavy lifting, so to speak. I would focus on the strongest pillar with the problem I chose to target. Afterwards, I would focus on the second strongest pillar, and so on and so forth. If I fixed the strongest pillar first, it was like this fixed pillar made the job easier each step of the way, or do I dare say possible. It strengthened the whole body to make it easier to fix the weak pillar when it was *its* turn to be fixed. So, this concept I call **strongest to weakest.** I know, not very original, but I don't think it could summarize it any better using any other words.

For example, the target is the large intestines. They are the weakest of the areas being affected by whatever it is. The other two areas being affected by the same problem were the lungs and small intestines. The main goal was the large intestines via the route of small intestines and lungs.

3. Deep, NOT Wide

The next concept is closely associated with this same process: ***deep, not wide***. I would like you to picture a pillar as the Grand Canyon with its many layers of different sedentary materials. When I focused on the strongest pillar, I would try to go through as many different layers as possible in a batch neutralizing session. I would look to see what would come to the surface by continuing to dig in the same spot. Whatever happened to be in the layers I was able to neutralize on the strongest pillar was not an issue on any of the other successive pillars for the next twenty-four hours. I did not have to do anything in order for it to happen either.

When growing a batch, the more I was "holding," the deeper I was going, and the less my detox organs had to do so they could focus on the root problem.

What did this look like at a homeopathic office visit? The first solution usually wasn't the solution. Holding the first solution for ten minutes would usually reveal what was underneath—assuming I was not currently holding anything. What is underneath is closer to being the real problem at this part of my journey. Because of this, once I figured out DISH, I always came to my appointments with different remedies or Good Guys taped to me or in my sock. It enabled my doctor and I to get down to business quicker in our search for the real problem.

4. The Root Is the "Gatekeeper"

This is the item I held so as not to have to hold anything else. The Gatekeeper is a big target with many things attached to it. If I'm holding it, my body is able to work on everything else combined with it without having to include this big guy. What I hold, I don't work on. But holding it does trigger everything connected to it. It forces me to work on those things. This Gatekeeper could be a Bad Guy or a Good Guy.

Bad Guy

- If the body is trying to fight two Bad Guys at once, holding one lightens the load to allow the body to focus on just the other one.
- Alternating back and forth between which Bad Guy I was holding enabled me to gradually be strong enough to fight the two Bad Guys together.

Good Guy

- Holding the Good Guy prevents the Mixing Point from happening.
- Holding the Good Guy could also make it easier to let excess or tainted Good Guys leave

(for example, cortisol), so the body will make more.

5. **The Gatekeeper Could be a Mimicker**

Sometimes I didn't need to necessarily know who the Bad Guy was (though doing so would make batches easier to figure out), but I needed to figure out what it was mimicking. It was more important to know what Good Guy was being affected than to know who the Bad Guy was.

This is a little complicated. Sometimes it is hard to differentiate a Mimicker from a grouped Good Guy/Bad Guy combo. But the good news is it doesn't really matter. Through the process of elimination, the truth is revealed. In Chapter 8, I will explain the three types of batches in which this Mimicker could be the Gatekeeper. I started with the easiest type of batch, heterogeneous. If it didn't work, I would proceed to the next type, homogeneous. If this did not work, I would try the third type, Mimicker. One of those, so far, has always worked.

Eventually, as my body and mind became familiar with these concepts, I just started asking up front what type of batch it was. Bearing in mind, every item in a batch is a unique unit. Each unique unit could be a batch in and of itself. I call this nesting.

Personal Examples

I learned how to control the amount of work my body needed to do by controlling my environment. I would need to avoid triggers and hold onto Gatekeepers. If I was at home or a place where I'd be staying put for a while, my environment would be changing less. I wouldn't need to hold as many items. But if I was to go someplace, I knew my body would be introduced to many other frequencies. Because of this, I would hold more items. By doing this, my body was able to focus on keeping the new frequencies I was being exposed to from becoming a problem.

I also learned that avoiding electronics and radiation during my weakest time of the day enabled me, for the most part, to be around them the rest of the day with just holding Gatekeepers or Good Guys.

By learning how Bad Guys behaved and the very elementary knowledge of the locations of organs and meridians in my body, I was able to start making connections. For example, I had severe leg bone pain for years. I found out the heel is correlated with the large intestines. I had been working some time on trying to find and correct the problem in my large intestines. It was so long ago, I don't even remember why, but I decided to tape Super Enzyme on my right heel only. It caused the pain to go away overnight. Whatever my body was trying to remove was taking Good Guys with it. This just let the Good Guys stay.

It predominately stayed gone. Occasionally it returned with far less intensity. I was able to be proactive though. I determined which Good Guy was needed and taped it on. Done and gone.

Thought to Ponder

Triggers

Many hair dyes contain a chemical called para-phenylenediamine, also called PPD. Some people are allergic to this chemical.[52] They need to find PPD-free options. I was reading the warning label on one such option. I found it interesting how it stated that, though it did not contain PPD, if someone is particularly sensitive to PPD, they should avoid using this product because they may have a reaction to it. Interesting. Is this a resemblance batch from a DISH trying to allow something harmful to leave the body? The dye with PPD missing had enough other ingredients similar to the PPD dye that the body saw it as an opportunity to try to remove what caused the reaction with PPD in the first place.

- Is it because all the other ingredients of the previous reaction are also present?
- Was this a close match to an equal equation, which, in turn, made the body try to fight and remove the PPD from the past?
- Is an allergic reaction just the trigger to get the ball rolling?
- If the Bad Guy is never triggered, will it always be there?
- Did we poke the bear as the saying goes?
- Should we even poke the bear?

---

[52] Ngan, Vanessa. "Allergy to Paraphenylenediamine." DermNet. August 2018. https://dermnetnz.org/topics/allergy-to-paraphenylenediamine.

  - If I wanted to get out of my cage, I needed to get the bear to get out of my way. However, just any way wouldn't work. I wanted to survive the encounter. The more I know, the better the chances of survival.

Batches

Are we already trying to control batches without realizing what we are doing? Does our body's desire to be well affect decisions we make without us realizing it is the reason we are making the decision in the first place?

- ***Hoarders***
  - Are they tied to their objects on a frequency level?
  - Are these objects Gatekeepers for them?
- ***Loners***
  - Are they trying to control how many new frequencies they are exposing themselves to?
  - Are they unknowingly fighting for self-preservation?
- ***Clothing***
  - When I stare at the clothing in my closet thinking *what do I want to wear today* does the color subconsciously matter?
  - Does the material my favorite clothes are made of make me like them?
- ***Disliked Food***
  - Is there a reason this food is not liked?

- Are you allergic to this distasteful food or does it trigger the loss of Good Guys?
- Does your body know on a subconscious level the food is bad for you?
- Is your body trying to get you to not hurt yourself?
- Does removing the danger cause you to now like the food?

The trigger is a chance for the body to remove the Bad Guy with less work—whether it is safe or not.

Conclusion for Chapter 6

If we avoid the problem, will the problem go away on its own? Or will it always be a hidden problem to come back and haunt us in our old age in many different ways? I think it depends on two things.

1. The status of our DISH, working or not working.
    - Working DISH—nothing is required to be done.
    - Broken DISH—need to create a manual DISH to make progress.
2. The type of batch the problem created.
    - Heterogeneous: possibly self-correcting
    - Homogeneous and Mimicker: need to be reprogrammed

Assuming we are dealing with a broken DISH, we are now at the point to combine all this new information. I know up to this point we have covered a significant amount of new information, new vocabulary words, new concepts, and principles. This chapter concludes the section of understanding the system. Reading the instruction manual is always different than doing it. However, it is necessary in order for you to understand the ideas in practical situations, which I will share with you in the next half of the book.

For now, let's keep in mind all the information up to this point.

Learn the system, then work it to our advantage.

Summary of the First Half of the Book

1. The functionality of DISH is a huge factor in our well-being.

   a. DISH works in conjunction with both the lymphatic system and the immune system.
   b. A working DISH prevents chronic inflammation.
   c. A DISH can be automatic or created manually.

2. DISH has two jobs.

   a. Protect the body.
   b. Sort what the body encounters.

3. There are two types of people.

   a. A working DISH—protecting and sorting is automatic.
   b. A broken DISH—protecting and sorting needs to be done manually.

4. Avoid the chain reaction.

   a. Be cautious during the Point of Saturation to avoid the Mixing Point.
      i. Good Guys need an exit to avoid being grabbed up with Bad Guys into the lymphatic system.
      ii. Good Guys and Bad Guys become grouped causes two problems.
         1. Body rejects the Good Guy(s) with the Bad Guy.
         2. Or body refuses to reject the Bad Guy because of loss of too much Good Guy.
   b. Prolonged misinformation will cause missing information.

   c. Once misinformation and missing information are both present, the vicious cycle begins.

5. Know how the invisible system works.
   a. Understanding how DISH worked enabled me to mimic it.
   b. The DISH worked regardless if it was automatic or manually done.
   c. Keep in mind the four concepts about players in this system.
      i. Triggers
      ii. Frenemies
      iii. Pathways
      iv. Cycling

6. Know my part in this invisible system.
   a. Be the strongest energy field.
   b. Remember the five principles.
      i. Batches
      ii. Strongest to Weakest
      iii. Deep, Not Wide
      iv. Gatekeeper
      v. Mimicker
   c. Control the Workload
      i. Vary the Gatekeepers I hold.
      ii. Strategically introduce Triggers.

7. Remember DISH is just a hypothesis.
   a. I am sharing what I have observed.
   b. I am sharing what I have learned.
   c. I am sharing what I have done.
   d. I am sharing what has worked for me.
   e. I do not know if it is true for everyone.

In the next half of the book, I will get into how knowing what I have shared with you so far enabled me to fight back. I enacted a process I've called Altering Fields to Enable Recovery (AFTER).

Section 3

How I Made This Invisible System Work for Me

CHAPTER 7: A MANUAL DISH

I did what my body should be automatically doing until it could do it again on its own.

Opening Story: L-Aspartic Acid Experience

I know my doctor can only prescribe for me based on the information he knows and is taught in order to have the titles he does. I know I was walking on shaky ground, but he was at least hearing me out. I needed to figure out a way for him to see what I was trying to explain. I had been praying about it and trying to figure out how to show him. I did not expect it to be during this next appointment, but it was, and it worked. He saw it firsthand. He continued to see it in successive visits as well, once he realized what I was showing him.

It was my normal visit. I would have typed out a page of all the pertinent information I had observed or figured out since my last visit. Each visit I usually narrowed down my problems or concerns to the two main areas I wanted addressed. There were many more issues than that, but I know I only had a short amount of time to convey my thoughts, and I didn't want to get sidetracked.

As usual, I quickly read off my sheet of paper as he took notes. I understood many principles at this point. For example, the more items I needed to hold, the closer I was getting to the main problem. The main problem seemed to almost always be a Good Guy being copied by a Bad Guy. It didn't really matter who the Bad Guy was, but what did matter was who the Good Guy was.

I wanted to find the Good Guy, but he wanted to look for the Bad Guy. Understandable. This is the protocol. But I wanted to do it backwards. He grabbed his vials and pointed out the many toxins I was testing positive for. I told him, "I know." I grabbed my bag out of my purse and showed him all the vials I was holding. I was holding over twenty different items, fourteen of which were Bad Guys. Here is the kicker—ALL of the toxins he said were the problem were in the purse. I saw the shocked look on his face. I explained how batches were like triangles, and I needed to find the top piece. If I found the top piece (Good Guy), all of these other Bad Guys would be a nonissue shortly.

I don't remember why or how, but I told him I suspected it was L-Aspartic Acid. It was. It worked. Within 48 hours, I no longer needed to take all of those vials with me everywhere I went. By just keeping L-Aspartic Acid in my energy field, the rest became a nonissue. Daily I sprinkled a tiny bit on my head and put the pill in my sock. Eventually, I no longer needed to do that either.

A question you may be wanting to ask me is, "Did you take any?" The answer is yes. I had been taking it for months in a combined form with other amino acids. However, this was not enough. Holding it in combination form did not work either. It needed to be isolated. It also needed to be outside of my body for forty-eight hours for the reprogramming. Afterwards, I took it orally for about twenty days. This was enough. I no longer need to take it. My body had reprogrammed. It was able to balance out.

Overview

I'll admit, in the beginning of this crazy journey, it just felt like a big, huge guessing game. But I pressed on and I started to notice patterns. Many patterns. Patterns that enabled me to realize what my body was doing. It confirmed my belief that what I was doing manually was something the body was supposed to be doing and wasn't. Because my body was not sorting, I did the sorting for it.

Sorting Is Sorting

The concept difficult for me to grasp in the beginning was how holding a Bad Guy worked the same way as holding a Good Guy. I concluded sorting was sorting. I needed to go through stages of dealing with the Bad Guy. As I was manually doing this sorting, the body still knew who the Good Guys and Bad Guys were. It had no need to grab up the Good Guys unless it was forced to—by them **taking the wrong road (because the road was blocked)** and being grouped with a Bad Guy.

1. Separate Bad Guy from other Bad Guys by holding all other Bad Guys except for the one I was targeting. This was just holding them back to target one Bad Guy at a time. The body somehow knew what to do.

2. The next stage is when I needed to hold the Good Guys. By holding the Good Guys, I was giving them an exit to prevent them from being grouped up. The body would stop rejecting beneficial nutrients.

Regardless of whether a Bad Guy or a Good Guy was being singled out, the reprogramming of the misinformation worked. I was helping my body to hold onto the nutrients/hormones it needed to become healthy again. To have a working DISH.

Grasping What This Meant

Earlier I had realized everything could be broken down. The same principle applied both ways. If there were two Bad Guys, separate them. If it was a Good Guy and a Bad Guy, the natural tendency would be for the Good Guy to be left alone. It only would get grouped with the Bad Guy if the roads were blocked. Holding these Guys constituted the same principle but for different reasons. Comprehending the significance of how small I could break it down eventually enabled me to neutralize the difficult problems.

For example, If I was able to break the Bad Guy down into seven separate pieces, I could target it in a manageable size by holding six of those pieces for fifty hours. I would then swap the current missing piece with a different piece for the same duration until I had done all the pieces. I was training my body to recognize each component. So, when I just wasn't strong enough to tackle a big Bad Guy, this gave me the extra help I needed.

The requirements of what to do depended on what was happening in the body. How the batch was made, what type of batch it was, and what was in the batch were all factors that needed to be included. Realizing I was dealing with four different scenarios revealed why there were inconsistences. But finding a way to get the body to accept or keep the nutrients always helped me to progress further.

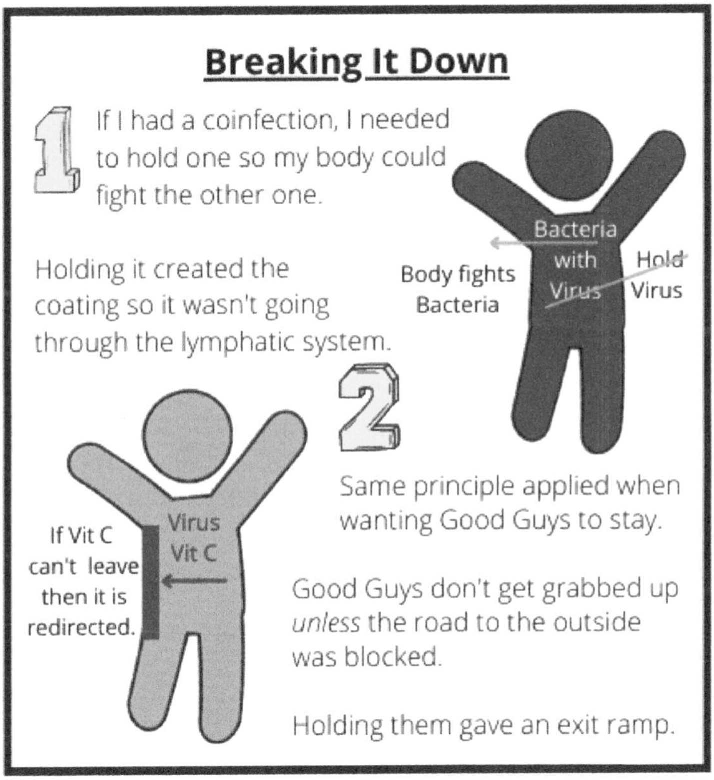
Breaking It Down
1
If I had a coinfection, I needed to hold one so my body could fight the other one.
Holding it created the coating so it wasn't going through the lymphatic system.
Bacteria with Virus
Body fights Bacteria
Hold Virus
2
Same principle applied when wanting Good Guys to stay.
Virus Vit C
If Vit C can't leave then it is redirected.
Good Guys don't get grabbed up *unless* the road to the outside was blocked.
Holding them gave an exit ramp.

Realizing the Significance of the Problem

I want to keep this very simple. Keeping DISH in mind, we want the outside to equal the inside. If the body is sorting, it is automatically doing this. If the body isn't sorting, it is looking for assistance to do the sorting for it.

Let's look at tuberculosis again. The tuberculosis vaccination is grown on egg.[53] So, tuberculosis and egg are connected (exposure). Because tuberculosis is tied to egg and the body needs the nutrients in egg, the body doesn't try to get rid of tuberculosis. When egg is consumed, the combination of tuberculosis with egg is a closer match. It is also the needed Good Guy. So, the body tries to act on tuberculosis. Sound crazy? Does it really? On WebMD.com, guess what food tops the list of foods to avoid for asthma? You guessed it: egg.[54]

Could this be part of the reason why? I think the body saw the consumption of the Good Guy (egg) as an opportunity. Unfortunately, it didn't have enough of those nutrients in the egg to get the job done. The body started fighting. It continued fighting until it ran out of Good Guys. The body retreated. Meanwhile, the Bad Guy had been provoked and

---

[53] IEEE Pulse. "New Vaccine-Manufacturing Methods Are Moving Away from the Egg." IEEE EMBS. 23 February 2021. https://www.embs.org/pulse/articles/new-vaccine-manufacturing-methods-are-moving-away-from-the-egg/.

[54] WebMD Editorial Contributors. "Foods That Can Trigger Asthma Attacks." WebMD. Reviewed 11 August 2021. https://www.webmd.com/asthma/guide/food-allergies-and-asthma.

was still provoked. (Picture a yappy little dog who won't shut up even after the confrontation is over.)

This idea is not far-fetched. Allergies are being corrected by giving the protein allergen to the person in small doses.[55] What if the reason this works lined up with DISH? The deficient Good Guy is getting enough reinforcements. Is allergy free really just trigger free? Should we look at everything backwards now? I don't know. I still have many questions.

The body looks for opportunities to

remove the Bad Guys.

---

[55] ScienceDaily. "Can Food Allergies Be Overcome with Scheduled Small Doses of Allergens?" Science Daily. 21 April 2008. https://www.sciencedaily.com/releases/2008/04/080417111254.htm.

Topic 1: What I Learned About Batches

Since everything is connected, everything is in batches. Different batches act differently. How a batch behaved depended on how it was formed, if anything was missing from it, and what type it was.

1. Batch Formation

When I say batch formation, I am referring to when the batch began. How did they become connected? The number one thing to remember here is EVERYTHING is connected, and everything needed to be singled out. Knowing how batches were formed made it easier to find the Guy(s) I was looking for.

When looking at the individual items, keep in mind it is not like a fork in the road. It is more like a spider web. A batch can very easily have been formed in all the ways I will mention. It just helped me to know where to start guessing. I know, guessing—not very scientific. But knowing how batches are formed made it more like an educated guess, which technically is the definition of a hypothesis.

A. *Exposure:* I was exposed to the items at the same time.

- **For example:** Styrofoam and coffee.
- **What this means:**
    - Look at the history of when the same Bad Guy was present at different times during my life.
    - What other Bad Guys may have been around at this time?

- Remember, a Bad Guy could be something that seems harmless (favorite toy—made of plastic).
- Could be an external factor or an internal one.
- **External:** Objects in environment.
- **Internal:** If it was an emotional time, include cortisol and/or adrenaline as an item in the batch.

B. ***Proximity:*** A Good Guy became attached to the Bad Guy just because they were on the same battlefield.

- **For example:** collagen and rheumatoid arthritis.
- **What this means:**
  - Protect against misinformation happening during times of inflammation.
    - ✓ What area was experiencing inflammation?
    - ✓ What Good Guys were needed there?
    - ✓ Hold those Good Guys.
  - Enable detox organs to maintain levels of Good Guys to keep doing their job.
    - ✓ If kidneys or liver are working overtime, I taped the Good Guys they needed on them. Sometimes preventing unnecessary loss is enough and the supplements didn't need to be taken.

- ✓ If I was low on a particular Good Guy, what organs needed that particular Good Guy?

C. *Resemblance:* The items were like each other.

- **For example:** kerosene and gasoline.
- **What this means:**
  - Similar Bad Guys tended to group together. If I was working on a virus, I was probably working on more than one.
  - Mimickers of Good Guys are usually found here.
  - Same Good Guys are needed to fight similar Bad Guys.

2. Batch Status

The second way of identifying a batch is whether or not all things were included in it. This factor affected how a batch behaved.

A. Complete batch: All Bad Guys that needed to be included were included. Progress was made. Eating would not cancel the batch. In a complete batch, the batch only needed to be done one time—meaning two batch neutralizing sessions in a fifty-hour period.

B. Incomplete batch: One or more Bad Guys were missing. They needed to be included in order for the batch to proceed. Sometimes it was difficult to figure out what was missing. A sign that something was missing was when eating something made my DISH go down. It canceled the batch, and the procedure would need to be repeated again immediately.

C. Canceled batch: I have noticed this occurring on five different occasions. The trouble with a canceled batch was it would make my shield go down. I would need to start over in order for my DISH to continue working properly.

1) If I cut the batch neutralizing session short, it would be an incomplete batch and my shields would go down.

2) I forgot to include something during the batch neutralizing session, which caused it to be an incomplete batch.

3) The batch became too big. An allergen triggered the batch to grow. This would result in a backup of Byproduct and/or POOP the body would get overburdened with.

4) I was around an energy field stronger than myself.

5) My energy levels—be they minerals or hormones or whatnot—would drop too low. It would be like an electricity brownout. If the power dimmed too much or blinked off and on, the shield would become compromised and need to be rebooted.

All of these are very similar in the fact that my body just couldn't handle the load it was given. I needed to only give my body what it could handle.

3. Batch Types

By knowing what type of batch I was dealing with, I could reprogram my DISH! Each type of batch had to be treated differently. By doing the required batch protocol, I would be able to get my body to accept the Good Guys while removing the Bad Guys. The supplements would be effective for me. My body would now successfully do what wouldn't work in the past. I could start eliminating the Bad Guys without hurting myself so much (chronic inflammation gone).

The only way I have been able to do this is through the process of elimination. The hierarchy is as follows:

A. Heterogeneous—A group of Bad Guys distinguishable one from another. (Think salsa... I could pick out the parts I don't like to eat, but it won't necessarily be easy; but it is doable.)

B. Homogeneous—A combination involving a group of Good and/or Bad Guys in a batch that is unable to become smaller by separating the Bad Guys from each other. The Bad Guys have become *changed* to where they can only leave as a single unit. (Think mayonnaise... good luck trying to separate the egg from the oil; it isn't going to happen.)

C. Mimicker—A Bad Guy replicating an essential nutrient or hormone the body needs. The body is having a hard time distinguishing the difference between the two. (Think identical twins... they are the same but not really.)

If the protocol for a heterogeneous batch didn't work, I would try the protocol for a homogeneous batch, and so on. I will explain how each type is dealt with in Chapter 8. But for now, realize by understanding there are three types of batches, it explained why, when I thought it wasn't working, it actually was. I just wasn't using the correct method.

4. What Finding Items in a Batch Looks Like

Here is an example of a partial batch of one I needed to work on. Keep in mind the more I included in a batch, the deeper I was going in finding the root of the problem.

Before we get into this example, I want to point out a few things.

A. Mixing Point Danger Zone

Back in Chapter 5, I explained the Mixing Point Zone. It is important to keep in mind potential proximity challenges to avoid hindering the process of this batch. By knowing what nutrients were at risk of being mixed, holding them, too, would prevent this from happening. Prevention is much easier than correcting. Where was the battle taking place? Which Good Guys were going in to help? The end goal was to stop losing Good Guys and to send in the reinforcements where needed to prevent them from becoming mixed with the Bad Guy.

B. Other Background Information

This is a compilation unique to me, which is factored in to the following chart. It should hopefully help you to see my thought process easier.

- For me, Rubella = Lortab = Egg. (Resemblance.) It does not mean it is the case for other people. It was just a pattern I noticed for me. Our DISHes are unique to each of us.
- I am assuming it is rubella. If the answer to the question was no, I would keep asking similar questions until I had a yes to start with.

- I had seen a homeopath for over three years at this point. I had many remedies on hand from what she had suggested.
- I also had many bottles of different supplements from trying to get well for years.

Once all the items were together, I proceeded with sway testing, keeping in mind the different ways batches are formed.

	Information I Have	What I Would Ask Myself	Items I Would Include
1	Coughing & rash: This rash looked similar to when I was told I had rubella in the past.	Ask? Is this rubella. Yes	Resemblance Items: Homeopathic remedy for rubella, Lortab pill from past surgeries, egg
2	I had rubella in the past. My mom had rubella. I was vaccinated for rubella.	What were other things in my environment during these exposures? Gather all yes items.	Exposure items: Christmas tree, dog, medication, carpet, cleaning solution for carpet, etc. My mom talked of getting a shot when she had rubella. (Cortisol? Antibiotic?) Egg, oxytocin, needle, Band-Aid, gloves
3	My lungs are being affected. Detox organs needed to fight the virus.	What are the Good Guys my lungs need? Gather all yes items.	Proximity items: Collagen, omega, copper, vitamin D, etc.—whatever I get a yes for

Information I Have		What I Would Ask Myself	Items I Would Include
4	When the virus dies, it kills the cell and dead virus is now in the system.	What will help with the Byproduct of rubella? What will help flush the virus out of the system?	Virus detox Doctor recommended supplements & water

5. Growing a Batch

This spot here is A BIG DEAL. This is where it gets complicated. I think most people's bodies do these batches automatically. Mine did not. This is a process of adding in more Bad Guys—in groups or one at a time—to the already existing targeted Bad Guy. The body will identify the groups of Bad Guys as complete sets that also needed to be neutralized.

What takes place during this time is one batch will be completed at the same time a new batch will begin. The batch isn't over with, though. Picture if you will a relay race. The baton has been passed to the next player, but the race is still going on. It will always go on. It is supposed to be an automatic system in the body complementing the immune system.

It is easiest to see this example by using colors.

For example, my target is red.

- I begin with only red.

- When I add yellow to the batch, I now need to neutralize...
  - ✓ Red
  - ✓ Yellow
  - ✓ Orange (Yellow with Red)
- I would then add blue to the batch. Now I need to neutralize...
  - ✓ Red
  - ✓ Yellow
  - ✓ Orange
  - ✓ Blue
  - ✓ Green (Yellow with Blue)
  - ✓ Purple (Red with Blue)

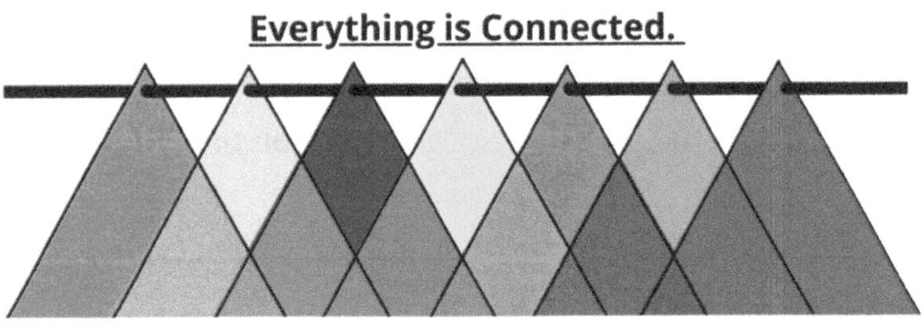
Everything is Connected.

A **color** can't be removed until it is released from all other colors first.

Note>> Each group (color) is considered a Bad Guy in and of itself.

- I would look back and look for ways the different colors are related to each other. I would notice all the colors (red, yellow, and the new color, blue) together made brown.
- Brown is now my new target. So, once this neutralizing session has taken place, instead

of needing to hold red, yellow, orange, blue, green, and purple, I just needed to hold brown.

If you look at the diagram of triangles, growing a batch was working my way up to the Kingpin. By the time I reached the Kingpin, I had neutralized as many triangles beneath it as I could. It was best if the Kingpin let go of all the triangles after they were neutralized. Otherwise, there was too much byproduct for the body to deal with and the lymph roads would get blocked again. This is why we start with the smallest triangle and work our way up. (*Going deep* would be trying to find the triangle with the most overlapping I can handle.)

If there was an exact match, it appeared to prevent any byproduct from being made. It just canceled. Hence, the closer the match before the removing of the Kingpin, the less Byproduct present (aka the less work organs needed to do).

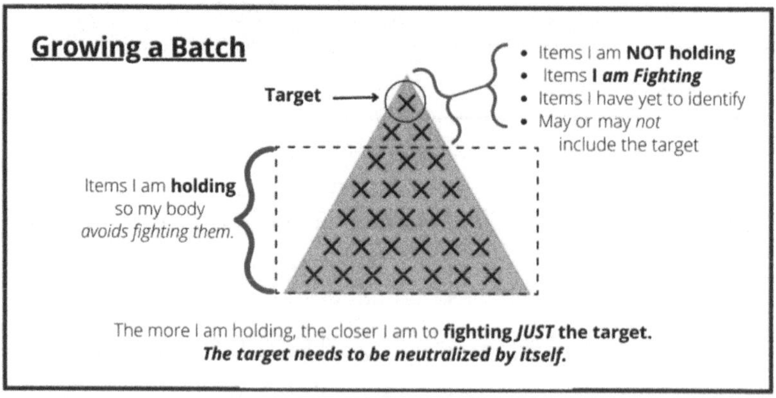

6. When to Target a Batch

Because of the meridian clock, different times of the day targeted different pillars. When targeting a Bad Guy, I needed to be aware of which meridian was the strongest one with the Bad Guy on it. If possible, I would then need to start my batch during this designated time. The batch would take a total of fifty hours to complete. I needed to *cycle* through this meridian window twice, once for the meridian and once for the organs associated with them. This fifty-hour chunk of time neutralized the Bad Guy I was targeting. Remember, I didn't make these rules up. These are just observations I have seen over the past decade.

Note: I would do a procedure during the strongest meridian clock. It took twenty to ninety minutes. Afterwards, I could go about as usual just holding what was required until the procedure needed to be repeated twenty-four hours later.

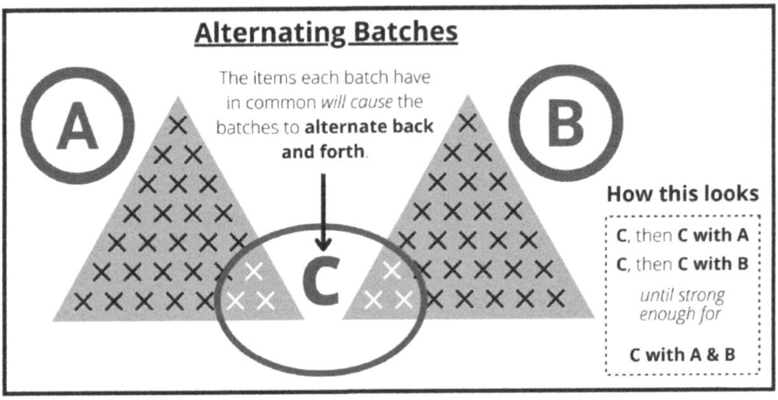

7. Alternating Between Batches

Another process I noticed was the body usually worked on more than one batch at a time. When it did this, it would look similar to the following diagram.

I would know this was happening by the alternating every few hours of what items I was holding. It would also reveal itself by observing the grouping of the supplements I needed to take. Each grouping would be consistent for the same Helpers each one needed. The groups would need to be taken with a span of time between them. These Helpers would associate with one group of supplements needed to fight A and the other group for fighting B.

This alternating is allowing the body to regulate the workload at a manageable size. Once strong enough, it will tackle both together.

This alternating batch would do whichever protocol was required for the type of batch each one was. Since two batches were involved, it required four days total instead of just the two.

Topic 2: How I Did It

The next chapter will go into detail about how each batch needed to be treated differently. In this chapter there were some basic things I did regardless of what type of batch it was.

1. Ongoing Requirements

A. Be the Strongest Energy Field

The most important part here was to make sure I was the strongest energy field around. This is incredibly difficult to do in the modern world. Yes, in the beginning, I sadly admit, it meant no computers, cell phones, or television for me. Knowing what I know now, this sabbatical may have been avoidable.

I have since learned scientists say electromagnetic hypersensitivity (EHS) is a self-diagnosed symptom that they think doesn't exist. Two to five percent of the population claims they are affected by it.[56] If we just considered the developed countries and looked at the low side of their populations, we are talking about over two and a half million people who feel effects from electricity. The reason given for no valid claim is because they believe other physical or physiological symptoms are at play. I feel so sorry for those

---

[56] Neuert, Michael R., MA, BSME. "Are You Sensitive to EMFs?" EMF Center. Last accessed 27 March 2023. https://emfcenter.com/are-you-sensitive-to-emfs/#:~:text=From%20the%20studies%20so%20far%2C%20it%20is%20estimated,as%20%E2%80%9CElectromagnetic%20Hypersensitivity%E2%80%9D%20%28EHS%29%2C%20%E2%80%9CElectrosensitivity%E2%80%9D%2C%20and%20similar%20terms%2A.

who try to seek help here and are blocked like this. I agree this EHS may not be the root problem, but I disagree about it not being there.

- It being there prevented my body from working on the other challenge.
- My body was busy protecting itself from this stronger frequency.
- In my weakened state, my body couldn't shield itself from electricity and sort my environment, and process out Bad Guys all at the same time.

Because of this, electricity was causing my shield to go down. I wasn't the strongest energy field. I was unable to work on maintaining my health. Yes, I was being negatively affected by the electricity. I didn't see this as an illness in and of itself. It was just another Bad Guy. It was basically another warning light on my health dashboard. With that being said, a Bad Guy is a Bad Guy. If it was food doing this, it would be called an allergic reaction. I think it should be looked at as a co-infection. Please, can we call it what it is? I prefer it over weirdo...

Regardless, I had to avoid electricity and anything else I was allergic to—food or environment. I wanted my body to be focused on the main problem, even if I didn't know what the main problem was yet. I didn't want it busy fighting electricity and allergies. This involved me needing to be continually aware of my surroundings.

During this phase for me, I was looking at my body as a sinking ship. Drawing on the knowledge of my practitioners was important. I needed to plug the holes. I used homeopathic remedies, essential oils, acupuncture, human growth hormone shots, a chiropractor, herbs, and whatnot. Whatever I could get to work to buy me time to figure this out.

B. Focus on Equal Sign

This would involve making sure the outside of my body equaled the inside of my body. I would hold whatever supplements or medication I was taking. By doing this, it would cause my body to avoid working on those and focus on the main problem. The same reason for avoiding allergens and stronger energy fields. I wanted the body to focus on the problem, nothing else. What wasn't in my energy field, my body fought.

It sounds ridiculous because it is so simple, but when I saw it as facilitating in my body's ability to sort, it didn't sound ridiculous at all. If my body can't stop rejecting the nutrients, how can I expect my body to have enough nutrients to heal and recover? When it came to medication, logically, I thought it would make it more effective.

C. Test Everything

Some people are surprised by how effective my sway testing is. Well, like everything else, it improves with practice. When I was so sensitive to my environment and my diet, I did not do anything without first sway testing to see if it would hurt me. I came to find out, for a period of years, I could only wear cotton or rayon. I was allergic to all other materials. Sometimes no zippers, sometimes no buttons. Everything mattered. Not cool, not fashionable, but necessary. For example, as I became stronger and polyester (plastic) was my target, I would need to wear it on just part of my body at a time. Wear polyester on my legs one day, on my arms a different day, on only my front or back on a different day. You get the picture. I did this for six months.

As I am sharing this, I think, *Who would want to do that? Nobody! Why should I tell anyone about this?* Why would I invite anyone into this CRAZY world of mine? And it always goes back to... it was the only thing that worked. I was desperate and I was willing to do the work. I saw improvement. I had hope. I had to press on. And yes, sometimes just knowing I had to play this ridiculous game daily would make me want to cry out in frustration.

I wasn't looking for an easier way;

I was just looking for a doable way.

D. Be Observant

I needed to be aware of my surroundings consciously so if my subconscious forgot something, I could mentally start listing off everything I could think of to help it find the connection it was searching for later.

For example, when I would have my teeth cleaned at the dentist's office, I'd scan my environment. Problems in my past consisted of radiation, vinyl, metals, and chemicals. So while I was sitting there, I was observing what each thing looked like it was made of. I made a mental note of the different smells.

Just by doing this one time, I realized as I was looking at the X-ray vest in the corner that it was made of lead. Aha, I bet lead is always tied to radiation. Progress forward for the next batch.

E. Add Routines to My Day

This goes back to testing everything. I needed to gear up for the day with what I needed. I would need to have a ritual I had to follow for eating. This ritual enabled me to remove all my food allergies, including gluten and dairy. (I know this is believed to be impossible for gluten, but...)

Soaking in the tub and going to bed at night is when I would make the most headway. I could keep my environment the same. I could be next to many things to go as deep as I dared. Granted, sometimes it felt like a snail's pace when I didn't yet know what I was doing. How much headway was I really making? Well, at least I was going in the correct direction. I could write pages for each one of these routines, but I do not want it to be the focus of this book.

2. Combining the Knowledge

As you recall, I mentioned there are three ways to describe batches. I combined my batch information with other knowledge. It was like putting a puzzle together.

A. Batch Formation

Understanding the three different ways they are grouped made it possible to narrow down the items in a batch.

1) Exposure
2) Proximity
3) Resemblance

B. Batch Status

By observing the behavior of the batch, I was able to determine if I was doing something wrong or making progress.

1) Complete
2) Incomplete
3) Canceled

C. Batch Type

Understanding there were three types of batches meant understanding there were three different methods to fix the problem.

1) Heterogeneous
2) Homogeneous
3) Mimicker

D. Other Knowledge Included

Like any new skill, trade, or hobby, it was important to not be overwhelmed by the massiveness of the task and knowledge. I tackled one small step at a time and just stayed consistent. I know very, very little about acupuncture and meridian points. I know very little about essential oils or all the other techniques out there on the fringe of alternative medicine. However, I did study the specific thing I needed to know about at a specific time.

1) Get good at sway testing.
2) Research on the internet.
    a. Learn how the body works.
    b. Learn about Bad Guys.
    c. Learn about Good Guys.

3) Study my past.
    a. Search for past possible Mixing Points.
    b. Search for connections to triggers.
    c. Search for potential missing information.
4) Consult with a homeopath or naturopath.
    a. Find Good Guys.
    b. Find Bad Guys.
5) Know my body.
    a. My strengths.
    b. My weaknesses.
6) Use meridian clock.
    a. Attack the problem during the strongest meridian clock time slot that has the problem I am targeting.
    b. Take it easy during the weakest meridian clock time slot.

3. Combining the Approaches

There is much talk of integrative medicine. Would knowing about how the DISH plays a role in health help it to be even more effective? When we think about necessary medication or vaccinations, we are concerned about the bad ingredients in them or their side effects. It's frustrating to work so hard on maintaining a healthy lifestyle and in one fell swoop be back to square one because I needed to go to the hospital or get an X-ray.

I know there are reasons to not want these toxins in our bodies. I agree. Sometimes, though, they are a necessary evil. But be warned, when the Good Guys are in with the Bad Guys... it is equally bad for those of us who have a broken DISH. We get them mixed up regardless of how good the

Good Guy may be. However, knowing there is a manual way to fix my DISH is a game changer. Holding the Good Guys on the outside of my body beforehand, and possibly for a time afterwards, could dramatically reduce the risk of side effects or errant programming from happening. I had to decide whether to do nothing and get the same results or do something different. But how could something so simple create such powerful results? *Right?*

Well, it does. When I went for my follow-up appointment for my appendix being removed, I could tell they were surprised at how well I could move and how symptom free I was. I also suspect she thought I was lying. But that was just a hunch. I have no doubt in my mind my progress was because I knew about DISH. I helped my body to do its sorting job when it was at its weakest.

When it comes to the approaches coined as unorthodox, we tend to think they don't work because we don't see results. By throwing the concept of DISH into the equation, the approaches worked better and usually within minutes. Occasionally it took three hours, an entire organ cycle on the meridian clock. I feel sorry for those people who start taking medication and see no results. They are told to *go on faith* that these might work eventually.

Understanding how the DISH worked enabled me to work it. What was currently going on with my DISH would enable me to be mindful of what approach I needed to be taking. When I was manually fixing my DISH, I incorporated the following:

- **Acupuncture points**—Enabled me to target one area of my body at a time.

- **Homeopathy**—Enabled me to include elusive items needed for a batch like viruses, poison, or other toxins.
- **Past medication**—What helped me hurt me; therefore, I needed to include them in my energy field so I could either work on them or what was underneath them.
- **Essential oils**—When unidentified Bad Guys are tied to the target, essential oils were more effective than homeopathic remedies. I also used them during alternating batches. I would use a homeopathic remedy for the target Bad Guy and an essential oil for the other Bad Guy.
- **Herbs & teas**—Sometimes removing Bad Guys caused damage; this helped the healing process when this happened. It also helped to occasionally strengthen the body.
- **Supplements**—Used significantly more on the outside of my body like a filter than on the inside of my body to increase the levels.
- **Magnets**—Sped up the healing process and kept the roads cleared when an intense emotion was associated with the target or an un-neutralized Bad Guy left.
- **Objects in my environment**—Used mostly in the beginning to remove all stragglers so I could focus on the main problem (target) at the time.
- **Self-talk**—Had the conscious mind teach or tell the subconscious mind what to do until it became automatic again.

- **Emotion Code**—Remove hidden barriers to recovering.
- **Colored glasses**—The color spectrum is an array of frequencies. When dealing with a resemblance batch with many items, sometimes using a color that is close to the frequency of the batch was very effective. I used these glasses or other items of color. Interestingly, I rarely wore these on my eyes. Most of the time I just wore them on the top of my head like a pair of sunglasses temporarily removed from my eyes.
- **And written reminders**—If my body was having a hard time remembering connections, I would write them down and read the note frequently over the next few days. Eventually, I just needed to tap the note to remind myself of everything on it. A type of speed reading for the subconscious mind if you will.

The secret to our health may very well lie in the ability to integrate all we have learned in all areas. How they are connected with each other. How they complement each other. One side says it's about the Bad Guys attacking us. Another side says it's about the Good Guys the body needs. Maybe DISH is what connects the two together.

For me, making my immune system stronger without a manual DISH made me sicker.

Topic 3: Patterns I Noticed

With the information I acquired over the years, I used many different things in order to manually mimic the coating I was missing from the surface of my skin. Sometimes I would need to hold them, sometimes I would need to have them next to me, sometimes I needed them on specific meridian points, and sometimes, if I was doing all areas of my body at once, I would need to take to the tub and put some in the water and soak in it to create the coating. Doing these things allowed me to function regularly.

1. Continually adjust DISH

This shield my body created changed from day to day, moment by moment. When I was very weak, I visibly learned the patterns I saw. I was able to take this knowledge and apply it to make progress. Anytime I changed my surroundings or

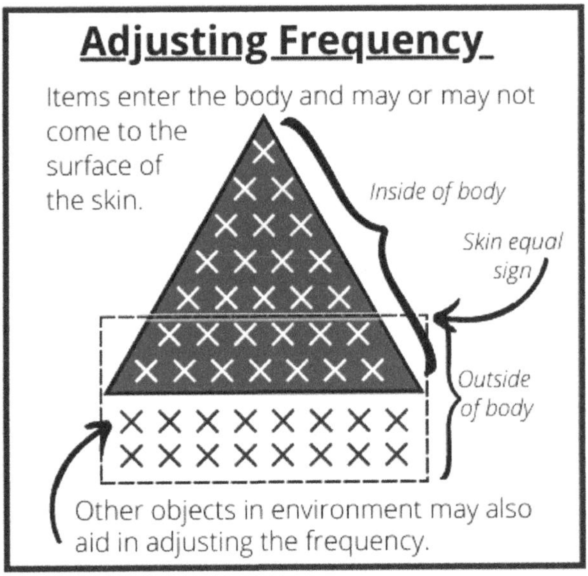

consumed something, my frequency should adjust. But it didn't. I manually had to do it. The amazing part was, by being aware of this lack of automatic sorting, and by manually sorting, I could be almost symptom free. The bad part was that I willingly fell into bondage to this manual sorting because it did work. Do it and feel fine, or don't do it and be unable to perform my daily tasks.

Some of this bondage was making sure I was keeping on the outside of my body anything going into it. If I forgot to do this, it would be like biking down the road and having the brakes suddenly seize up.

2. Closed Circuit

Here is a diagram of the earth's magnetic field. Notice the closed circuit. It was easier for me to grasp this concept if I looked at this energy field in a visible way. Instead of thinking of it as energy, I thought of it as water. With that in mind, this energy field was recirculating. It was not like a river just flowing out to wherever it wanted to go. It was acting more like a fish tank recirculating the same thing continually.

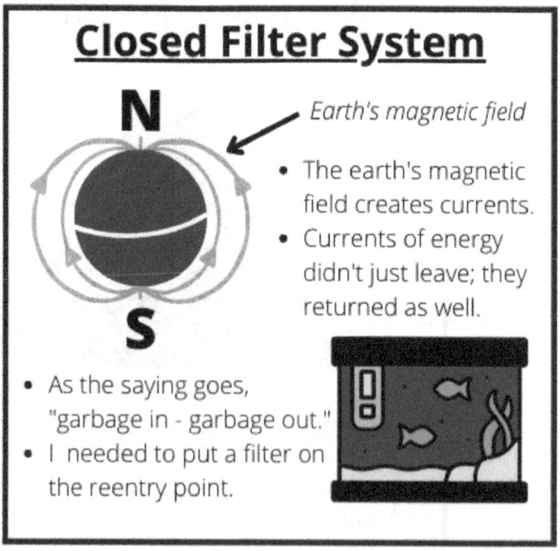
Closed Filter System
N
S
Earth's magnetic field
The earth's magnetic field creates currents.
Currents of energy didn't just leave; they returned as well.
As the saying goes, "garbage in - garbage out."
I needed to put a filter on the reentry point.

The water would not, could not, improve by just doing that. It needed a filter to stay usable.

Transferring this thought process to our energy field, I noticed sometimes I needed to constantly reapply my essential oils in order for me to feel the benefits. Well, that was frustrating, messy, and expensive. This is when I decided to place a small amount of essential oil on a tiny piece of a cotton ball and tape it either on a meridian point or the organ area. *Boom!* I have myself a filter. I did not need to continually reapply over a large area of my body all the time. This was very effective once a target had been neutralized.

However, it is different during the process of a batch neutralizing session. When a target was being neutralized, I would be focusing on one part of the body during its time of the day on the meridian clock. It would have to be the part of the body strongest at fighting the Bad Guy I was targeting. I would lie down in a neutral environment. I would place the appropriate essential oil in my belly button. (FYI: For food allergies, I used lemon oil unless it was egg, which required hyssop.) I would then lie there for twenty to sixty minutes depending on whether or not I was using magnets to *pull* the energy quicker. Once the pull of the magnet was gone, I would wipe out the tainted essential oil and reapply one drop of the same oil into the belly button. It was like step one cleared the area and step two did the work.

This was also true when I would have a homeopathic remedy taped on a spot on my body. When it was time to have it removed because it had *cleared* the area, I would need to apply some type of essential oil on the same spot. If I did not, it would not hold. I would have to re-clear the area again.

Clear the meridian, clean the meridian,

and then heal the meridian.

---

3. Signals

Depending on what time of the day I needed to strengthen my DISH by soaking in the tub to create a coating or when the batch neutralizing session needed to take place, I could tell if I was making progress.

- Growing a Batch: Batch was needed done on the strongest meridian.
- Releasing a Batch: Batch was needed done on the weakest meridian.

4. Time Frames

I noticed patterns as I progressed through batches. By being aware of how the DISH system worked, I was almost able to schedule it on my calendar to a certain degree. It also enabled me to plan my day somewhat ahead of time, which hadn't been able to happen before I figured this out.

Seeing the patterns enabled me to know when I would need to *do a batch neutralizing session* and when I could plan to *be hit* by the climax of a batch. At the climax of a batch, I would need to take it easy for organs to focus on doing their jobs. I noticed consistent time frame patterns. I was learning as I was going. I do not know if this can be sped up. I didn't make the rules. I just observed what was happening to me.

- Two, ten, or twenty minutes to neutralize one Bad Guy—in one place on the body—depending on factors involved at the time.
- Forty-eight to fifty hours to release the same Bad Guy, depending on when I started. I began with a batch neutralizing session. Afterwards, I held the main ingredient of the session for fifty hours. During this fifty-hour window, I would repeat the batch neutralizing session again on the same meridian clock: remember, once for the organ and once for the meridian. I would continue to hold the main ingredient for at least four days afterwards.
- Four, ten, twenty, forty, or sixty days before the release of the one Bad Guy (in one place on the body). It depended on how many other Bad Guys it was related to that hadn't been neutralized yet.
- Nine to fifteen months from the Bad Guy being neutralized in one place to the Bad Guy being neutralized in all places (aka released).
- Two to six years to being completely removed from the body.
- Hold supplement for forty-eight hours before taking.
- Take supplements four to twenty days in a row, then repeat every twenty to sixty days.

5. Repetitious Four Layers

The easy part is knowing it is all about equal signs. My body needed help to continually change its DISH to make the outside match the inside. The other easy part is realizing how batches work so I could determine if I was making progress or not. Still another easy part is most of the time just holding whatever I needed. worked wonders. The not so easy part was being patient as I worked through each layer repeatedly for groups of batches.

These groups of batches usually contained three main batches, which were usually attached by a Kingpin. I have worked through this process three times so far. Each time I finish the fourth layer, I can feel a significant boost in my energy, and what I need to hold drops down to one to three items. As I work through the layers, sometimes I will end up needing to hold over thirty items until I have figured out the Kingpin. But once I have, they become nonissues and remain nonissues.

My system needed a reset. I needed to start with the easiest job first and work my way up.

A. Layer One: Protect, Prevent, and Proceed Mode (3Ps)

I don't have exact percentages here, but I would venture to guess at least eighty-five percent of the time I was in this 3P Mode. However, this layer would focus on bigger issues every time after going through all layers and coming back to this point for the next Kingpin. I would also be stronger so I could fight the next *bigger* Bad Guys.

During this layer, I would be holding what I did not want my body to reject if it was a nutrient. I would be holding Bad Guys too—referring to co-infections. This would make my detox organs' job easier. Holding these items in my energy field consisted of striving to go deep and not wide in my batch. The more I held, the deeper I was going, the closer to the root problem I would get. And the less work my body had to do. Only when this was not working did I need to advance to the next layer. If I chose to just maintain, I could stay here. If I wanted to improve and flip the switch back, I would have to proceed to the other layers.

If all a person does is this level, our bodies have a chance to focus on why we are taking the Helpers (supplements & medication) in the first place. Our immune systems can deal with the problem by itself without needing to include the Helpers too. If I'm wrong, nothing should happen. Nothing should change. No harm, no foul. But if I am right, progress is made, and isn't that why we are taking our supplements and medication in the first place?

B. Layer Two: Train the Body

A Good Guy(s) and a Bad Guy(s) were stuck together. I needed to manually do the sorting for my body in order to retrain it. It still blows my mind how effective this is. How I trained my body for misinformation is in Chapter 8.

Even though the training steps only usually took fifty hours, I would technically be knocked back into Layer One for nine to fifteen months per Bad Guy. However, the number of batches I could be working on at this level could be a massive quantity. They didn't need to be one at a time once they were past this point.

C. Layer Three: Focus on the Target (Triangle Tops)

Each triangle was a batch in and of itself. The bigger the triangle, the bigger the batch, the more items involved. In this layer, it seemed like the body always wanted to focus on three unique triangle tops at a time. (See page 145.) Ideally, once the three big triangles were cleared, the Kingpin could then be safely removed with the least amount of health issues. Remember, the closer the match, the less the detox organs had to work, the easier it was on me as a person.

D. Layer Four: Remove the Kingpin (the Rod)

The only way I was able to determine I was dealing with a Kingpin was when I had neutralized a number of big targets (big triangle tops), and in spite of doing this, I was still needing to hold many items. It could become very discouraging at this layer. The key to maintaining high spirits here was to know, once the mimicked nutrient or hormone was identified, it was a BIG DEAL. The dam would be breached. There would be a flood of toxins. This is why I want as many batches (triangles) neutralized as possible.

When I finally realized the pattern on this layer, I would be excited when this was happening. I learned once the Kingpin Good Guy was figured out, I would have two days of reprogramming my body, two days of die-off, and then a big jump in the improvement of my health for several months as long as I continued to hold the Good Guy Kingpin.

So far, for me, the Kingpin has always been a Bad Guy mimicking as a Good Guy. This made the Kingpin difficult to recognize. Sometimes I would be needing to hold trace amounts of over fifty different things until I figured out what the Bad Guy was mimicking. But once I did, I only then needed to hold this single Good Guy. Holding the Bad Guy would not work. Occasionally, I would be able to figure out who the Bad Guy was, which made growing the batch easier. Other times, I never knew who he was, but it didn't stop my progress. It just made the growing of the batch a little more difficult, but not impossible.

Personal Example

How soon is this progress? I don't know. It depends. Sometimes it is instantaneous. Sometimes it is a gradual acceleration. And sometimes it is just not going backwards. For me, I was just aiming for not going backwards and the other ways happened.

I am going to use the example of a virus. The virus is going to be a part of a simple batch. Nothing is connected to it anymore. "All the same-colored liquid is at the top of all the tubes" (Colors Game Analogy, Chapter 6.) This is what it looked like when I manually did my DISH's sorting job.

	AFTER Approach	Symptoms & Procedures
1	Chain is off.	Energy low. Feel sick. Maybe coughing.
2	Find Problem.	Sway test to narrow down what and where the problem is. It's a virus everywhere. (It is at *the top of all the tubes* in the analogy.)
3	Take Helper to fight Problem.	I take and hold elderberry liquid to fight virus.

	AFTER Approach	Symptoms & Procedures
4	Problem being worked on.	I feel better. Body is fighting virus and winning. The body is making cortisol to fight the virus. Organs are working hard and *sweating*. All goes well as long as *the roads aren't jammed up in preexisting traffic or too much organ sweat.*
5	Problem starts to be destroyed.	Virus is dying. Blood cells are being destroyed and replaced.
6	Problem creates Byproduct.	Dead virus starts to build up on body. Organ sweat also builds up.
7	Problem and Byproduct of problem build up.	Body now needs to remove virus and virus Byproduct. *Roads* are getting crowded.
8	Chain falls off.	Load becomes too much. Symptoms return. Or viral infection starts to become a bacterial infection. Byproduct and Problem become combined making *roads* even more crowded.

	AFTER Approach	Symptoms & Procedures
9	Byproduct and Helper are now part of the problem.*	Helper's alternate exit (going to the surface of the skin because it was considered harmless) is blocked. He is caught up in the traffic jam. He is now redirected and grouped with Problem and Problem's Byproduct.
10	Hold Helper and Byproduct to keep fighting virus.	What I am holding provides the exit for everyone except the target. It allows the body to focus only on the targeted Bad Guy. The virus is separate from *the group*.
11	Start fighting Problem again.	As long as holding virus Byproduct and Helper, able to keep taking Helper and focus only on virus. Might possibly need to hold proximity Good Guys as well.
12	Start winning against problem because body is stronger than first time the problem was confronted.	Before chain fell off, progress was made fighting the virus so organs are stronger now.
13	Batch grows, so start doing combinations of the three (Problem, Helper & Byproduct of Problem).	Problem of the combo still circulating. Want to teach body to leave Helper alone and to fight Problem alone and with Byproduct.

	AFTER Approach	Symptoms & Procedures
14	Body learns how to fight Problem with and without Byproduct by alternating them within my energy field.	As body becomes stronger, periodically keep Byproduct out of energy field. Body needs to be able to train itself to fight both together since sorting system isn't doing this yet. Periodically place Byproduct back in energy field when combo becomes too much for the body.
15	Problem gets fixed.	When DISH is working and load is not too much for system, the body does the sorting itself so it no longer needs to be manually done.
16	Body heals.	Body is doing its job. It is also healing from any damage caused. The body starts doing a system check. It goes through and removes all released unattached Bad Guys. Removing them boosts the immune system.
17	Fixed Problem boosts immune system.	The body is able to level up. It is stronger, so it thinks it can fight more difficult problems.

	AFTER Approach	Symptoms & Procedures
18	Immune system fights the next Problem alone.	This boosted immune system starves the parasites that were feeding off the inflammation from the virus pulling out Good Guys with it.
19	The lymph roads start to get bogged down.	New Byproduct was introduced. Parasite die-off.
20	Try to help immune system before chain falls off. (Assist in sorting.)	Holding supplements I'm currently taking and holding supplements of the type the targeted organ would need protects Good and Bad Guys from combining.
21	Keep moving forward.	Finish fighting aftermath of immune system boost.
22	New Bad Guy(s) is revealed.	The body will continue to do its sorting job. The DISH will stay up until it comes across something not released yet. New target found.
23	Repeat cycle again.	It may seem like I need to hold so many things. But not really. Only a trace amount is needed. Sometimes I used a spray. When it was the Kingpin, I only needed to hold one to three things. The more I did need to hold, the closer I knew I was getting to a major Kingpin. **

*The interesting thing here is that holding the Helpers before starting to target Problem worked, but holding the Byproduct beforehand did not. I had to wait at least twenty minutes before holding the Byproduct. Evidently the body needed to do something first.

**When I targeted the L-Aspartic Acid Kingpin, it was the only thing I needed to hold for months. But working up to this Kingpin, I was holding over thirty different things in order to function properly. But hey, they all fit in a small bag that just needed to be near me, and doing this let me function properly.

Action Steps Summary

- **Sway Testing**
    - I have included an appendix in the back of the book to explain how I managed to get good at sway testing.
    - I believe this is just a communication link between our conscious and subconscious mind.
    - My body needed to understand the questions I was asking.
- **Stop the Leaks**
    - Find the weak areas.
    - Tape what I needed on the weak areas.
    - Think: Putting a filter on a closed circuit.
        - Supplements
        - Essential oils
        - Homeopathic remedies
        - Any object
            - This could be anything in my environment.
            - If it is toxic, I place it in a container and avoid direct contact with my skin.
    - Having the filter in place prevented the need for reapplication.

- **Be the Strongest Energy Field**
  - Avoid excess or unnecessary electricity or radiation.
  - Be continually aware of when I felt a dip in energy and observe what happened just before or forty-eight hours before it happened.
  - Manually adjust my environment accordingly.
- **Avoid Known Allergens**
  - This included diet and environment.
  - If my body was working on fighting the allergen, it had fewer resources available to fight the targeted problem.
  - Want the body to focus on only one problem at a time.
- **Keep the Good Guys Around**
  - Learn what Good Guys the injured part of my body needed.
  - Keep those Good Guys in my surroundings, ranging from on my person to within hands' reach to just being in the same room.
  - This prevented a proximity batch from forming.
- **Prevention Is Easier Than Fixing**
  - I always held the supplements to allow the programming of the lymphatic system to happen.

        - When prescribed a new supplement, I held it for forty-eight to fifty hours before taking it for the first time.
        - When taking the Helpers, hold for ten minutes before or for twenty minutes after taking them.
        - I did the same with my food.
    - If the problem is avoided, there is no problem to fix.

Conclusion for Chapter 7

The idea that holding something in one place would enable the entire body's shield to go up may seem a little difficult to wrap your head around. Instead of looking at the item as being what is creating the shield, look at it as the shield is already there. It has a leak. Putting the needed object into my energy field is just the code for plugging the leak. It is inserting the information, so it can circulate throughout the shield. Because the body should naturally be continuously doing this frequency adjusting, it does get tiresome doing it manually. It is also liberating. It is getting me unstuck from poor health.

Creating the DISH manually enabled me to maintain my health. It enabled me to function normally again. But improving my health did not occur until I also fixed the misinformation and the missing information in my body. For the correcting of missing information, I saw no real harm or danger. For the misinformation, I will freely admit it was sometimes not safe. It depended on the type of batch and the behavior of the Bad Guy being attacked.

It is like opening a hole I was unable to clog up again. What caused the flipped switch was still there. The Bad Guy could cause it to flip again. I wanted the Bad Guy removed from my body. Doing so was purposefully trying to trigger allergic reactions so I could adjust my DISH to reprogram the problem, to separate the good from the bad. These were not light loads because the vicious cycle I have told you about was still circulating.

The next chapter will explain how I did this reprogramming of the lymphatic system based on the type of batch I was working with

.

CHAPTER 8:

CORRECTING THE MISINFORMATION

Reprogramming the lymphatic system

Opening Story: The Importance of Sulfur

During this stage of my recovery, I was actively looking for triggers; those nuisances that needed to be reidentified in the lymphatic system. They were hidden. They were not obvious. For me, it required researching random nutrients and body parts on the internet, looking for connections. The body needs so many things to function properly: vitamins, minerals, amino acids, good bacteria, HCL, enzymes, and more. With amino acids, there were the essential (body could not make) and nonessential (the body could make) ones. Lying among them were also sulfur-containing amino acids.

How far does misinformation need to be broken down?

As far as it needs to.

Now, before you think I must be some smart person, I want you to know I do not understand the details of what amino acid falls under what category and why. I just read on the internet the list of sulfur-containing amino acids:

methionine, cysteine, homocysteine, and taurine.[57] All of which were recommended to me in the past.

I took this information, dwelled on it, and went into the kitchen to prepare supper on our gas stove. Guess what? Since gas is odorless, sulfur is added to it so leaks can be detected before causing significant injury. Sulfur. Sulfur with petroleum products. Petroleum products from daily life and from exposure to contaminated Camp Lejeune water. Is this a problem for me? Maybe. I knew one way to find out. I went into the living room and dug through my boxes of remedies until I found sulfur—also a remedy that was recommended to me in the past. I placed it in my pocket and kept it there.

Forty-eight hours later, almost to the minute, sulfur was freed. When this happened, I became suddenly and severely dizzy and nauseous. I needed to lie down for twenty minutes. When I got up again, I took a dose of sulfur. It was the only dose I needed to take. I was very tired the rest of the night but felt much better the following day. Now, if I keep sulfur in my pocket when I'm cooking, I do not need to take Methylsulfonylmethane (MSM). If I forget to have it on me

> MSM is a huge source of sulfur, which is a critical component of collagen. This may help promote the tightening of skin fibres on a cellular level, helping to stop cellulite from developing. Again, more research is needed to confirm this, however, many MSM users report seeing noticeable benefits from taking MSM powder to tighten the skin.
>
> www.thebircherbar.com.au/blogs/musings-muesli/what-does-msm-powder-do
>
> **What Does MSM Powder Do? The Key Health Benefits**

---

[57] Brosnan, John T., and Margaret E. Brosnan. "The Sulfur-Containing Amino Acids: An Overview." National Library of Medicine. Last accessed 27 March 2023. https://pubmed.ncbi.nlm.nih.gov/16702333/.

while cooking, I would become fatigued. I would need to take a dose again.[58]

Makes no sense and sounds almost superstitious UNTIL you understand batches. If I had this sulfur in my pocket, my body would reject the petroleum and leave the sulfur behind. This action was my manual DISH being adjusted. My body could now identify the sulfur from the sulfur gas. Holding this sulfur was the frequency the artificial DISH for my body needed in order to be able to allow the petroleum to leave. If it was not there, it would reject the petroleum with the sulfur until it became too low on sulfur. It would then just HOLD the petroleum in my body. It would not try to remove it anymore. I would become "toxic."

Since prevention is so much easier than correction, I chose to keep holding this sulfur whenever I was around the stove when it was on (or the gas fireplace). My current life prevented me from being able to remove those toxins from my surroundings permanently. This was my work-around. It has worked well for me.

Overview

In this chapter we are going to finally delve into the nitty-gritty of these batches I keep talking about. I guess you could say there are three types of batches, plus a bonus batch.

1. Heterogeneous
2. Homogeneous

---

[58] Ogdon-Nolan, Darcy. "What Does MSM Powder Do? The Key Health Benefits." The Bircher Bar. Last accessed 27 March 2023. https://www.thebircherbar.com.au/blogs/musings-muesli/what-does-msm-powder-do.

3. Mimicker
4. Nesting

Each one of these batches acts differently. How to use the knowledge of these batches is what made it possible to remove my Bad Guys and keep my Good Guys.

First, know that all three types of batches can be formed in the same three ways: exposure, proximity, and resemblance. All batches can also be at a different status: complete, incomplete, and canceled. What differentiates the batches the most is their interaction with other items in the batch: heterogeneous, homogeneous, Mimicker.

All batches followed a similar process to remove the Bad Guys. The details of how to follow the process depended on the type of batch. Allow me to summarize the basic process for all batches in the following analogy before we look at each one individually.

What This Looks Like:

ANOTHER GAME ANALOGY

The Playing Field

The best way to describe what is going on is to look at it like a video game. The first levels are easy, but each level I progress through will either include more enemies or more aggressive ones. I don't know if it's possible to just "skip" to the end of all the levels and battle the final challenge to complete the game.

The body may need to make itself stronger first by passing all the other levels, removing all other Bad Guys. That way, all my focus can be directed at only the "final challenge" of the game. At least, that is how I had to do it. Does that make sense?

The Rules of the Game

- **To Win:** Eliminate all Bad Guys while keeping the Good Guys.
- **How to Accomplish This Goal:** Separate the Good Guys from the Bad Guys while keeping the chain on the bike (Bike Analogy Chapter 1).
- **Warning Whistle:** Inflammation, low metabolism, and candida are the brakes on the bike. It was my body's way of telling me to slow down or the chain will fall off again. The Good Guy has not been separated from the Bad Guy yet.
- **Objective:** In the simplest explanation, picture a fistfight. I cornered the Bad Guy all by itself and started beating it up until I started getting in more punches than the Bad Guy.
- **Obstacle:** When his friends saw this, they tried to rush in to help him. The friends are the Byproduct in this analogy. These Byproducts started beating me up also. I could win against just the one, but not when I was being ganged up on.
- **Strategy:** I needed a way to prevent his friends from coming in to help. How did I keep this Byproduct at bay? I held the Byproduct in my energy field. (For example, homeopathic virus detox.)

It enabled me to battle only the one I was focused on. When I was done fighting the original Bad Guy, I then turned around and looked for the other "challengers." If they were minor, they usually fled. If they were more intimidating, they were next. (For example, stop holding virus detox. If I'm holding it, I'm not working on it.)

Guidelines: TWO GROUND RULES

1. **Everything Is in Batches**

Just as no man is an island, *no Bad Guy is independent of other things*. The key is to understand how batches are made. I needed to single out the Bad Guy from the rest of the items in a batch before I could start attacking it. For example, let us say I really love jelly beans, but I absolutely hate black jelly beans. I hate them so much that I always destroy every black jelly bean I see. Now somebody dumps a pile of jelly beans onto the table. Am I going to start smashing the black jelly beans with a hammer, or am I going to put them in a separate pile from the rest of the jelly beans before I proceed to destroy them?

The better I understood batches, the easier it was to break them down into smaller pieces. By doing that, I could single out a particular Bad Guy to target it.

2. **Avoid "Key Players"**

For me, these Key Players were the particularly harmful Bad Guys found in the Camp Lejeune water poison: benzene, radiation, plastic, and more. If I continued to encounter these Key Players, I would be adding batches to what I needed to fight before I could single the Bad Guy out.

So, I considered any contact with these Key Players as a step backwards. If it was a football game and we were trying for a first and ten, we just lost twenty yards. This is why it was so complicated for me. These Camp Lejeune Bad Guys consisted of some really Bad Guys. If they kept entering and leaving my energy field, it would "trigger" an exposure batch of some really harmful stuff, forcing me to have to deal with (fight off) all those Key Players together. There is more to it than that, but let's stick to the basics.

My Game Plan

Single out one Bad Guy at a time to eliminate. I started with egg. It was number two on the NAET list I mentioned earlier. It was also a known allergen for me. I had to avoid egg and all other allergens. Because of Camp Lejeune, this was particularly difficult. Benzene, plastic, and radiation are EVERYWHERE, in obvious ways and *in disguise*. Talk about a difficult task.

For example, it took me nine months to single benzene out from the rest of all the other items. (Basically, because it was in the ***Camp Lejeune water***, anything that came into contact with water was fair game for being part of this benzene batch. Ugh!) I was looking for parts of an exposure batch. I would take this information and start off with assuming it was a heterogeneous batch. This is where understanding how different batches work would come into play. The way I singled it out was by thinking of what else I was exposed to at the same time and holding them first. Holding them kept me from having to work on them.

Once I was strong enough to fight benzene, I needed to hold it in my energy field ALL THE TIME. For *two years*. When I was doing this, I was "growing" batches. I was tackling everything connected to benzene. By holding the benzene at this point, it enabled me to not need to fight benzene. It enabled my body to focus on the Bad Guys "connected" to benzene. Benzene was being prevented from joining the fight. (Holding this benzene allowed me to have regular energy throughout the day.)

Once my body was able to fight what benzene was connected to, and its combinations, I would periodically put benzene outside of my energy field. All those items I was holding to get to benzene would now be slowly removed one at a time from my energy field. Each one I removed had me fighting the item with benzene. Over time, as I countinued to remove each one, my body would proceed to target each one and their combinations of each other and benzene. (If we are lucky enough for it to be a heterogeneous batch.)

This went on for another two years. Sometimes I needed tea tree oil to help strengthen me to fight the batches. But I did all this benzene fighting before I realized that, for me, benzene mimicked TMG (trimethyl glycine). It is a rare nutrient that my thyroid needed in order to operate properly.[59]

---

[59] Dr. Christianson. "7 Rare Nutrients Your Thyroid Needs to Survive." Dr. Christianson. Last accessed 27 March 2023. https://www.drchristianson.com/7-rare-nutrients-your-thyroid-needs-to-survive/.

Once ALL the items in ALL the batches were neutralized, benzene was then a nonissue. *Neutralized*, if you remember from Chapter 5, is a term I concocted to mean the body is fighting and able to defeat a Bad Guy. It did NOT necessarily mean the Bad Guy was GONE from the body though.

For example, if benzene was the color red, and we finished getting rid of all the red, would it be gone? If there was the color orange someplace, then NO. Because red with yellow made orange. See? What next?

Train My Body

I realized I needed to reprogram the misinformation. I was dealing with a resemblance formation. I needed to separate the Bad Guy (benzene) from the Good Guy (TMG). I needed to hold TMG in my energy field for fifty hours and avoid consuming any TMG or benzene at that time. (This batch was a Mimicker batch, so it needed to be treated differently than the previous batch.)

Once I retrained my body, I was cleared to replenish my TMG levels and they would actually stay replenished, whereas before they would not.

If I noticed I needed to start taking TMG again, it was a clue the "chain fell off" again. Hold TMG again and keep moving forward.

So, as you see, this was/is no easy game to play. I would not wish it on anyone. But with that being said, it was/is worth it to me. It gave me my life back. The patterns and procedures are there. They consistently worked for me once *I figured them out.* The patterns are still working for me.

At this point I would like to say, "And that is how the game is played. That's it." But instead, I have to say the game gets even **more complicated**. Yes, there seemed to be an endless number of rules to follow to play this game. (There are homogeneous batches and nesting batches as well.)

I'm only participating because I had no other choice. But I also think the game would have been easier to play if it were not for SO MANY factors that were in my past. (Mainly the Camp Lejeune water contamination, several events that happened to my mom when she was pregnant with me, and living in two foreign countries during my childhood.) But that being said, with each new concept I figured out, my health always improved. I found the road. I hope to continue to smooth out the trail to make it easier to travel next time.

Key Point:

The type of batch determined the different procedure the body needed to fix the sorting.

Topic 1: Heterogeneous Batches

1. Description

A heterogeneous batch is the most basic batch. It is a combination of Good Guys and Bad Guys that are distinguishable one from another. Think salsa. The tomatoes, onions, and peppers could be picked out individually. It is always where I started. For a heterogeneous batch, the key takeaway is to give the Bad Guy permission to leave.

2. Personal Example: Peanuts

(**DO NOT DO THIS!** I am just sharing information.)

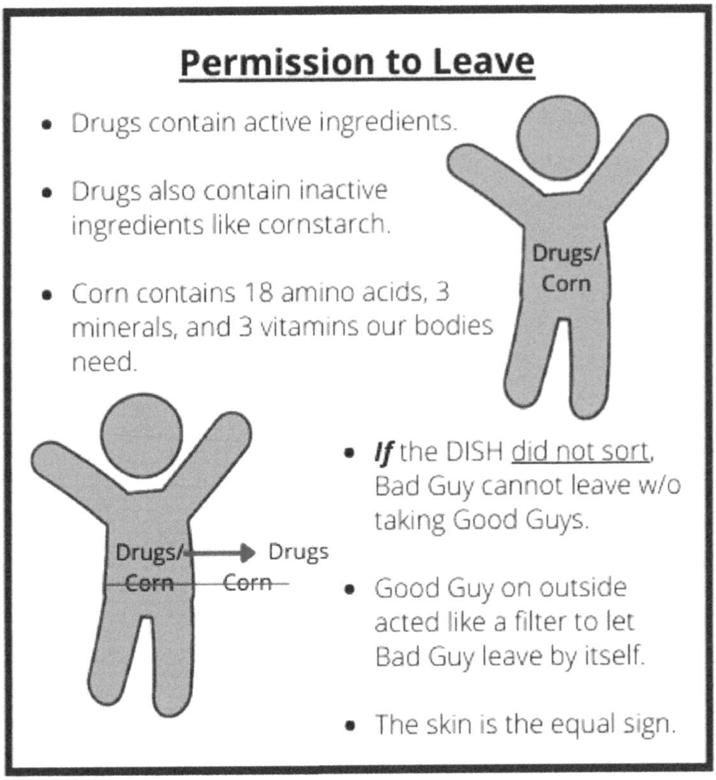

Permission to Leave
Drugs contain active ingredients.
Drugs also contain inactive ingredients like cornstarch.
Corn contains 18 amino acids, 3 minerals, and 3 vitamins our bodies need.
Drugs/ Corn
Drugs/ Corn
Drugs
Corn
If the DISH did not sort, Bad Guy cannot leave w/o taking Good Guys.
Good Guy on outside acted like a filter to let Bad Guy leave by itself.
The skin is the equal sign.

I had not yet realized the nutrient rejection connection when this occurred. We were living out in the country and the closest civilization was not even qualified as a town, really. It was considered a CDP, a census designated place. In fact, our closest neighbors were a gas station, a biker bar, a cemetery, and two churches. I kid you not.

Needless to say, I was eating lunch and had my first allergic reaction to peanuts ever. Among other symptoms, it was making it significantly difficult to breathe. My husband was home and a fire station was about two miles away, so I could get there quickly if it became worse. So, I decided to test my theory. I started putting all the homoeopathic remedies I had been working on in my energy field. Because of all my research, I knew there was a fungus common in peanuts considered to be a cause of cancer.[60] Because of this information, in this particular batch, among other things, was the homeopathic remedy asp fungus, different cancer ones, and variolinum. It worked.

I needed to avoid peanuts for the next year and a half. At the time, I slowly started building a batch around them. I now have no peanut allergies.

3. How to Identify This Batch

I would say probably over ninety-five percent of my batches were in this category. A common sign for when I needed to do this batch was if I would display symptoms of both too much and not enough of a Good Guy.

---

[60] Levy, Jillian, CHHC. "Aflatoxin: How to Avoid This Common-Food Carcinogen." Dr. Axe. 2 May 2016. https://draxe.com/nutrition/aflatoxin/.

4. How to Fix It

I needed to continually reprogram the body as my environment changed until the DISH started staying up automatically. The way to manually reprogram a heterogeneous batch is the same whether it is dealing with two Bad Guys or a Good Guy and a Bad Guy. The need to do it with two Bad Guys would be because the body wasn't strong enough to fight both at the same time. The need to do it with a Good Guy and a Bad Guy is because the Good Guy was being rejected. The same procedure worked regardless of which situation it was.

Normally, all I needed to do was hold the Guy(s) I didn't want to currently fight and take and hold what Helpers I needed. If, during this time, I continued to show signs of having too much and not enough of a particular Good Guy, I knew I would need to do a batch neutralizing session. It looked like this:

I would do a batch neutralizing session

only if just holding the needed item wasn't working.

---

5. What a Batch Neutralizing Session Looked Like

- I would grab an empty jar slightly filled with filtered water.
- I would take the two Guys and place a trace amount of each item into the jar and swirl or shake it.
- This gave me three items.

- I would sit with those three items in my energy field (about four to six inches from my body).
- I would sit there for a minimum of twenty minutes.
- I could not have anything come in and out of my energy field at this time or I would have to start over.
  - ✓ For example, a cat jumping on the table or a person walking by me.
- It took ten minutes to neutralize everything in my environment.
- It took the next ten minutes for the reprogramming.
- After the twenty minutes, it would then be like growing any other batch.
- I would slowly add additional items into my energy field, then wait.
- I would then start slowly removing them from my energy field.
- I would end with needing to hold only the Good Guy who was reprogrammed.
- I would repeat this twenty-four hours later on the same meridian clock.
- Slowly adding in the other items made it significantly easier on my body in the days to come.

When this process was done, holding the necessary nutrient/hormone was required for a long period of time (weeks/months). During that time—to make it easier on my body—I needed to periodically touch the batch I made for releasing the load.

6. How to Know If It Corrected

This batch neutralizing session helped my body to reidentify the different components. It realized what it could and couldn't keep.

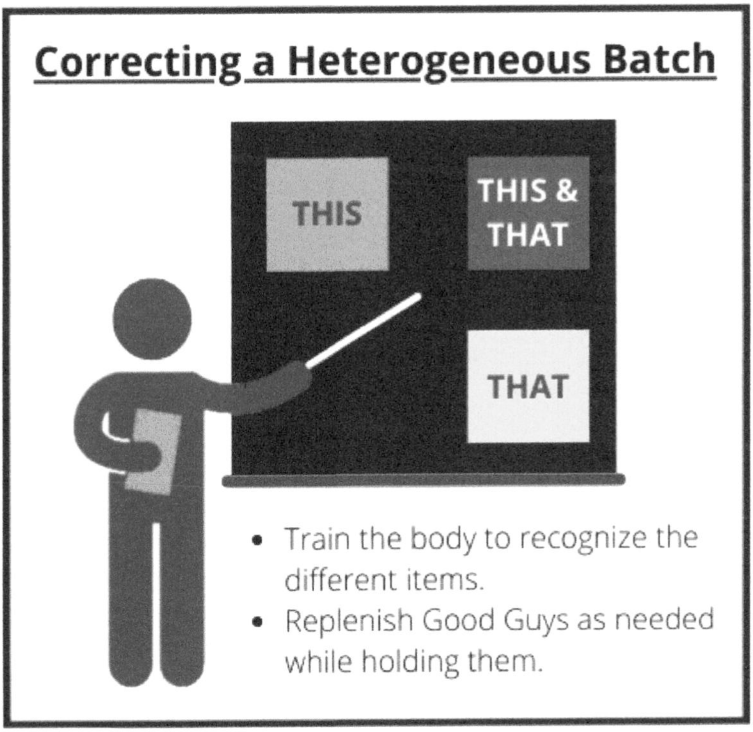

- About forty-eight to fifty hours in, I would need to take some of the Good Guy the batch was built around.
- Forty-eight to fifty hours after this, my body would start dumping the Bad Guy—toxin surge or parasite die-off would result (I needed to be careful).
- My nutrient levels would stay up for the targeted Good Guy.

It usually took about nine to fifteen months of building the batch around the Bad Guy target to complete it. My body rarely needed help during this time. Just a waiting game.

I think the heterogeneous batch is the only batch that can correct errant information automatically with a properly functioning DISH. When one of the two items is reintroduced, a frequency is made on the skin to do the reprogramming.

7. Key Takeaways

- Holding a Bad Guy(s) will lighten the load to where I could focus on one Bad Guy at a time.
- Holding a Good Guy gave the Bad Guy permission to leave without taking the Good Guy with it.
- The Bad Guy leaving will create a toxin surge about forty-eight to fifty hours later.
- The Good Guy staying will reduce how much you need to take to maintain proper levels of Good Guys.

Heterogeneous:

Instruct Bad Guy on how to get permission to leave.

Topic 2: Homogeneous Batches

1. Description

A homogeneous batch is unable to become smaller by separating the Guys (Good and/or Bad) from each other. The Guys have become *changed* to where they can only leave as a single unit. Remember, think mayonnaise. Good luck trying to separate the egg from the oil. Not.

It is fine if all the Bad Guys are bad, but if it has been bound to a nutrient or hormone the body needed, the body would end up attacking itself (chronic inflammation) when it was trying to remove the Bad Guy.

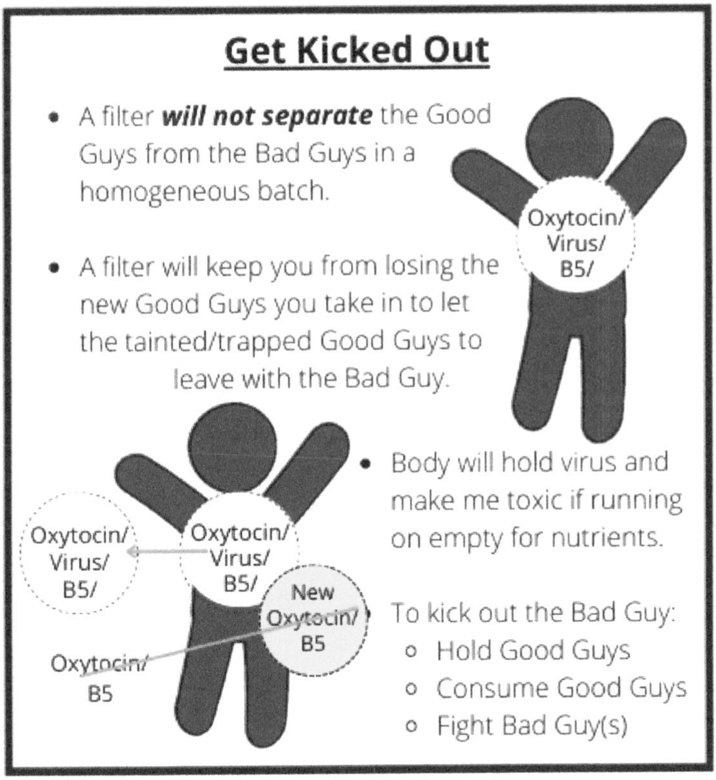
Get Kicked Out
A filter ***will not separate*** the Good Guys from the Bad Guys in a homogeneous batch.
A filter will keep you from losing the new Good Guys you take in to let the tainted/trapped Good Guys to leave with the Bad Guy.
Oxytocin/ Virus/ B5/
Body will hold virus and make me toxic if running on empty for nutrients.
Oxytocin/ Virus/ B5/
Oxytocin/ Virus/ B5/
New Oxytocin/ B5
Oxytocin/ B5
To kick out the Bad Guy:
Hold Good Guys
Consume Good Guys
Fight Bad Guy(s)

2. Personal Example: Good Guys Bounded to a Virus

Instead of permission to leave, we needed to just kick the Bad Guy out. The Good Guys stuck with the Bad Guy are not usable or of any use to us. Kick them out. In the process of doing so, the new Good Guys need to avoid the side road. Hold the Good Guy so there will be exit ramps for it.

For example, I had a virus I could not fight. I always became too weak to do anything about it. When I narrowed the problem down to oxytocin and vitamin B5 being attached to the Bad Guy, I could do this batch to get rid of the virus. I would hold the Good Guys and take small doses of them. I would also need to take something to fight the virus at the same time. By holding the Good Guys, the new Good Guys would not get grabbed up. By taking a Helper to fight the virus, I would trigger it to leave. It would take the tainted Good Guys with. It knew reinforcements were coming.

3. How to Identify This Batch

A homogeneous batch is usually the next step. These seem pretty rare. I have had fewer than a handful. This could be a group of only Bad Guys or a combined group of Good and Bad Guys. For this type of batch, the misinformation needed to be dealt with differently. This batch was more complicated.

The main way to know it was a homogeneous batch was if the batch neutralizing session did not work. The sign this was the case was if I was still needing the targeted Good Guy very regularly. Another way to know would be if taking a Good Guy or Helper lowered the levels of a different Good Guy significantly.

4. How to Fix It

The key takeaway was in order to have the Good Guys needed to fight the Bad Guy, we needed to kick the Bad Guy out while preventing the new Good Guys from being lost with the current wrong programming. Each individual component still needed to be identified. However, in order to remove it, all the good nutrients in the group needed to be taken to force the Good Guy–Bad Guy group out.

- **Just Bad Guys:** All Bad Guys needed to be included or the Bad Guy I forgot to include would hurt me. I had to fight both Bad Guys or neither.
- **Good and Bad Guys:** Consuming the Good Guy will trigger the group to leave, but by holding the Good Guys, the new Good Guys will not be lost. (Redirected to lymph nodes to be identified as Bad Guys.)

For example, while studying patterns of supplements I was taking, I suspected L-phenylalanine and tin (both Good Guys my body needed) were tied to a Bad Guy. If I took just L-phenylalanine, it would trigger me to fight the Good Guy–Bad Guy group. It forced the group to be pushed out. This would pull the tin out with the Bad Guy, lowering my tin levels and causing harm to my body. But if I took both supplements at the same time, the body would not be harmed and it would continue to remove the Bad Guy.

By putting these Good Guys in my energy field, my body would start holding the untainted Good Guys I was consuming. When the body realizes there will be a regular replacement for the tainted Good Guys, the rear guard (Car Analogy) would give the order that the tainted Good Guys were no longer needed. The Good Guy–Bad Guy combo would be rejected. It would now be safe to take what measures are necessary to permanently remove the Bad Guy from the body.

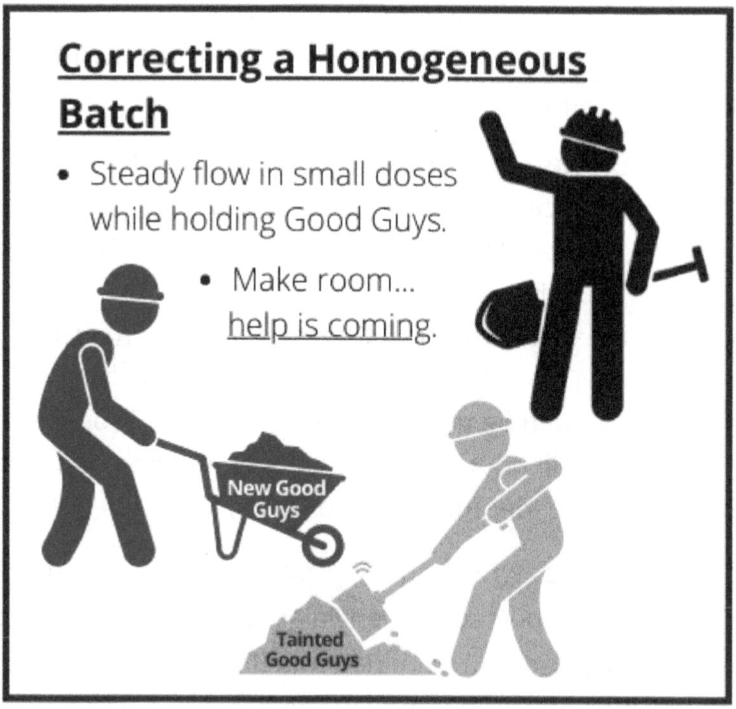

5. Getting the Body to Let Go of a Homogeneous Batch

- I needed to identify the Good Guy(s) being rejected.
- I would hold the Good Guys as continuously as humanly possible on my person for the next nine to fifteen months.
  - Once I needed to hold it for two years!
  - If holding a pill in my pocket instead of taking it kept my knees from swelling, fine with me. I'll do it.
- During this time, I would be taking the Good Guy(s) frequently. Duration was more important than quantity.
- It did not need to be a full dose—a trace amount usually sufficed.
- I would hold these Good Guys so they wouldn't be diverted. Only the Good Guys with the Bad Guy would continue to be diverted to the lymph nodes.
- Holding the Good Guy gave it an exit ramp to use. This holding was the manual DISH reprogramming my sorting system.
- I would fight the Bad Guy.
  - I would take supplements or use essential oils.
  - I would need to give my body a rest period for twenty-four hours to prevent losing too many Good Guys. (Stop taking the non-targeted supplements.)
  - I would next need to periodically place the Bad Guy Byproduct in my energy field.

- If the need for Byproduct showed up, it meant progress was being made.
- I was killing the Bad Guy and I only needed to keep the roads clear.

6. How to Know If It Corrected

Short answer, the body would start doing what it was unable to do before. What this looked like: I had a homogeneous batch of a virus combined with oxytocin and B5. If I held those two supplements on me, my body would now be able to fight the virus. It would be safe to help my immune system by taking elderberry liquid, vitamin C, and so on without it hurting me. My body was now fighting this virus.

I knew I was finally fighting this virus because the supplements I would now need to take were centered around this. I needed to remember when a virus died, the blood cell it was in died as well. I needed to make sure I was drinking plenty of water and focused on the supplements needed to make new blood and protect what organs were doing the work.

In order for it to stay corrected, I had to keep the Good Guy in my energy field continually and control the outflow of Bad Guys. It would now be safe for me to use what is called *binding* supplements to escort the Bad Guys out. It would also be safe to fight the Bad Guy more aggressively.

7. Key Takeaways

➢ The Grouped Bad Guy/Good Guy of a homogeneous batch is viewed as a single item. Since it has a Bad Guy, it is a bad item.

➢ Make the replenished Good Guys be identified differently than the tainted Good Guys.

- Replenishing Good Guy(s) was more about frequency than quantity.
- The body needed to know reinforcements were coming.
- Holding the Good Guy acted like a filter to enable the sorting.
- Don't want the tainted Good Guys to leave too fast.

Homogeneous:

The Bad Guy(s) needed to be slowly kicked out to maintain adequate levels of Good Guy(s).

Topic 3: Mimicker Batches

1. Description:

A Mimicker batch was hard on the body. It is when a Good Guy was unable to remain in the body because its seat was currently taken by a Bad Guy. The body saw the Bad Guy the same as a Good Guy. No matter how much Good Guy I would put in, I could not replenish it. The Bad Guy was refusing to be removed. I had to make a void in order for the reprogramming to work.

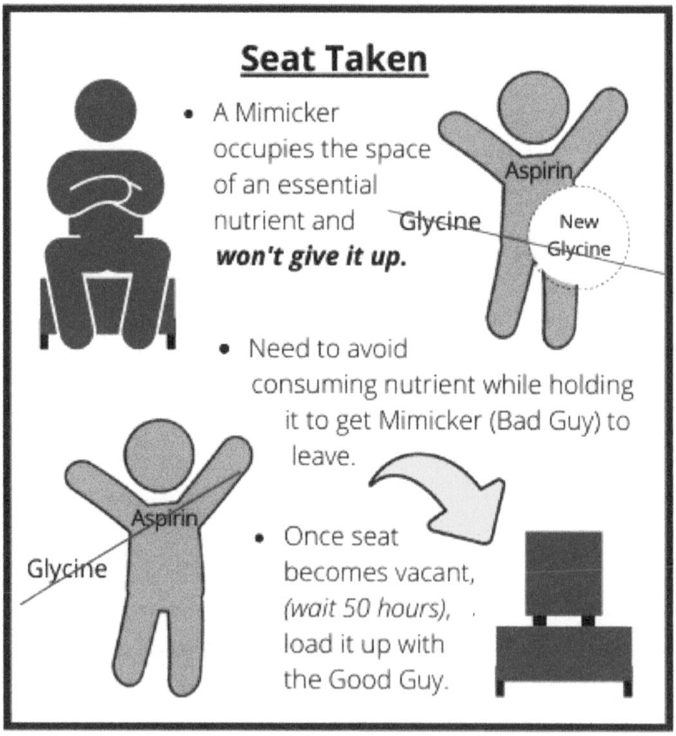

2. Personal Example: Bad Guy Was Mimicking L-Aspartic Acid

I had a suspicion the Bad Guy was a drug from surgery, but I could not *detox* it out of my body. Nor could I flush it out. However, when I realized what was being mimicked, holding the Good Guy for fifty hours while avoiding consuming it worked! Not knowing who the mystery Bad Guy was didn't matter. I just needed to know what Good Guy he was mimicking. Afterwards, I needed to front-load L-Aspartic Acid to fill the void created. I talked about this experience at the beginning of Chapter 7.

If the DISH was broken, recirculating false information would never make the information become true. Nor did recirculating it faster.

3. How to Identify This Batch

This was more like a one-on-one type of batch. Let's say we have this *space* in our body. This *space* is supposed to be occupied by a specific nutrient or hormone. However, a Bad Guy who is similar to the needed item is currently occupying the space. No vacancy. No vacancy caused two possible scenarios.

- **Hormone:** If the needed hormone's space was currently occupied by a Bad Guy, the body thought it did not need to make any more of the hormone. The body mistakenly thought it already had enough, even though it couldn't use the Bad Guy (or tainted Good Guy) who was being a squatter there.

- **Nutrients:** If the needed nutrient's space was currently occupied by a Bad Guy, the body thought it had plenty of the nutrient already. It would reject the mistakenly believed excess the body was bringing in.

Regardless of which scenario was happening, the body needed to be taught this was not the case. The body needed to reprogram the faulty information into accurate information. This is how I knew I'd probably stumbled across a Mimicker.

- I would be holding many items in order to feel normal.
- I would not be taking or holding any supplements to indicate I was creating Byproduct or making progress forward.
- I was like this for more than three months.

These were the hardest for me to identify because nothing seemed tied to them. They were more like squatters. They were occupying the space of a nutrient or hormone even though they were not doing the nutrient or hormone's job.

4. How to Fix It

The key takeaway is to avoid taking in new Good Guys while holding the Good Guy. This will force the Bad Guy out of his seat. For whatever reason, just holding the Bad Guy would fail to do the same job. Tried it. It didn't work. It had to be done this way.

Here is where the problem lies though. When I do this, there is a period of time when I do not have the nutrients needed for the body to function properly. I had to wait out the dumping of the FAKE Good Guy. When doing this batch, during the time leading up to the fifty-hour marker, I would feel a growing ill feeling coming on. I was creating the void. This may show up in many forms of what would be considered symptoms of being *too toxic*: nausea, dizziness, weakness, pain, and the like.

Dumping the FAKE Good Guy left a void—a void that needed to be refilled sooner rather than later. But I had to wait until he was done leaving the particular pillar I was targeting. This Mimicker can only be removed over time. It was like having two glasses of water. One full of clean and the other full of dirty water. First the body needed to know which glass was the clean and which was the dirty. (The fifty hours of holding.) After that, I just needed to dump some dirty water periodically, every time another pillar was reprogrammed to dump the Bad Guy. After each successive dump, I would take one larger than normal dose (but not exceeding recommended daily amount) of the Good Guy during the first two to six hours. This would be pouring clean water into the dirty water, diluting it—what I called front loading. This dilutes it over time until it is eventually all clean water. This periodic normal dosing of the Good Guy would be taken while holding them. I would continue to hold this Good Guy(s) for a very long time—twenty days to two years; it just depended on what it was. But trust me, I would know if I needed to hold it still. It was that obvious.

Look at holding this Good Guy as a type of filter to keep the Good Guy in. Remember, there are different stages of a batch. This forty-eight-to-fifty-hour period is the body identifying the Bad Guy. The end of this period is when it is neutralized. Twenty days later, it is released in one place. Over the next nine months to six years (for me, for egg), the body will systematically release and remove it from the rest of the body with just this "filter" in place. I would add and remove other Gatekeepers to regulate the size of this batch during this time period.

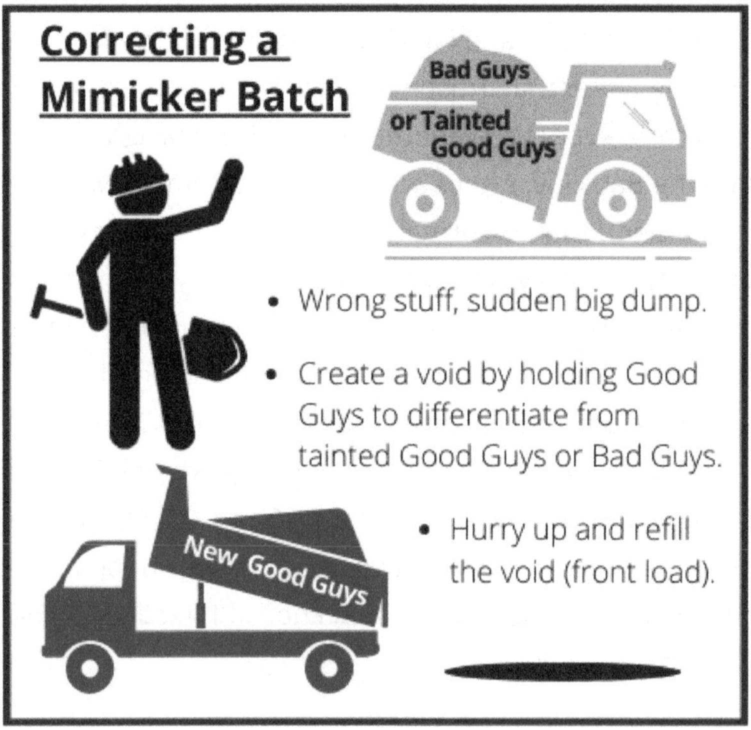
Correcting a Mimicker Batch
Bad Guys
or Tainted Good Guys
Wrong stuff, sudden big dump.
Create a void by holding Good Guys to differentiate from tainted Good Guys or Bad Guys.
New Good Guys
Hurry up and refill the void (front load).

Better a spot filled poorly than not filled at all.

The main significance of this batch was that a void needed to be created, then filled. It was hard on my body because, for a short time period, I had to operate on very low Good Guys while also trying to fight the Bad Guy who was just dethroned. This happened most during the first couple of releases of a Mimicker. After that, it is almost unnoticeable.

5. Getting the Bad Guy to be Dethroned

- I had to do research to find connections based on how batches are made.
  - Exposure
  - Proximity
  - Resemblance
- Even though technically it is a resemblance batch, sometimes it is only found using the other two methods.
  - Sometimes this took a long time.
  - Once found, if I didn't already have the Good Guy in my possession, I would acquire it.
- Hold the Good Guy for forty-eight to fifty hours without consuming it.
- The time frame was completed when I would feel the "hit." I would either be suddenly nauseous, dizzy, or feel the need to lie down for twenty minutes.
- Once the "hit" happened, I knew it was time to start filling back up with Good Guys.
  - The body will be significantly low on the Good Guy when the void is created from the Bad Guy leaving.

    - I usually had to front load the Good Guy with larger than normal doses for four to six hours.
    - This is when it is more about quantity than frequency.
    - The replenishing duration is shorter than a homogeneous batch.
- Usually happened in two stages.
    - First Stage: forty-eight to fifty hours later—one pillar was targeted.
        - If something else was connected to it, it took twice as long.
        - Once void was created, refill it.
    - Over next nine months to two years:
        - Need to continue to hold twenty-four/seven.
        - Each successive pillar would be reprogrammed.
        - Just holding the Good Guy allowed the body to do the rest.
        - If another "hit" was felt during this time, I would sway test if another pillar cleared and needed to be replenished.
        - The *hits* taper in intensity.

6. How to Know If It Corrected

The main way would be the *hit* happening and the need to front load Good Guys. If the hit did not happen, I would continue to hold another two days. It meant it was possibly an alternating batch (Page 179). After the front load, I would need to systematically take these Good Guys, for example, once every ten days. I would also be able to tell if I was still correcting by placing the mimicked Good Guy out of my energy field. I would feel the negative effects of it easily within five to thirty minutes. This was particularly frustrating after cleaning up for the day. I needed to as quickly as possible re-create the manual DISH I had just washed off if it wasn't in the water I was soaking in.

When the last pillar cleared, I would always notice something felt different but couldn't put my finger on it. I would ask my body if this was the final release. Yes.

7. Key Takeaways

- Holding the Bad Guy won't work.
- Need to hold the Good Guy the Bad Guy was imitating.
- Need to hold and avoid consuming the Good Guy for forty-eight to fifty hours.
- The time frame was completed when I would feel the "hit." I would either be suddenly nauseous, dizzy, or feel the need to lie down for twenty minutes.
- Once the "hit" happened, front load Good Guys.
- Take it easy for a few hours, allow body to flush out Bad Guys.
- Just holding the Good Guy twenty-four/seven allowed the body to do the rest.

Mimicker:

Needed to make the seat vacant for

the Good Guy(s) to be allowed to take the spot.

Topic 4: Nesting Batches

1. Description

I know, I said there were only three types of batches. This is true. However, I have included what I guess you would call a bonus batch. A nesting batch is basically what the name implies. It is a batch inside of a batch.

It isn't just a smaller batch. For me, it was always a homogeneous batch. For example, I needed to hold the supplements that were equivalent to chlorinated hydrocarbons—what is needed for the body to make lipids.

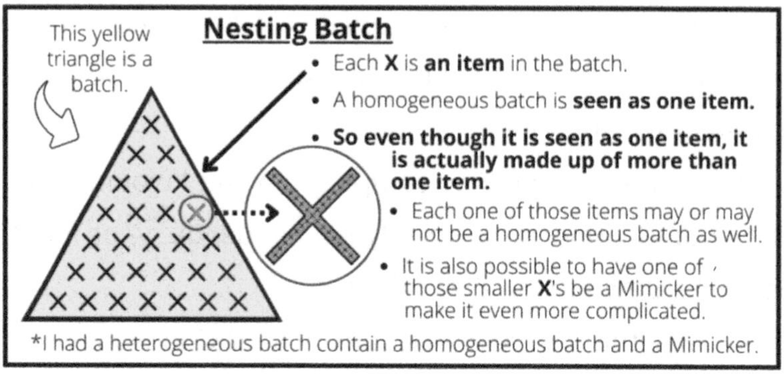

This was the Good Guy, but it had to be a combination (homogeneous batch) of Good Guys to make it A GOOD GUY. This Good Guy was nested inside of a batch involving pesticides and other items. Pesticides are chlorinated hydrocarbons—the Bad Guy Mimicker.

2. Personal Example

For me, oxytocin was the Good Guy of two Mimickers, Pitocin and chlorabutanol. Oxytocin was also part of a homogeneous batch I will share in detail in Chapter 11.

3. How to Identify It

If the other three types of batches did not work, it meant I was missing something. It did not *act* the same as a smaller batch inside of a larger batch. It *acted* more like a single unit. I needed to go deeper in search of what Good Guys were missing. For me, it meant I was getting closer to the finish line because of the harmfulness of the Bad Guys that revealed themselves. It will consist of two players.

- **Nesting Batch:** The main batch (the orange X shown below). This orange X would be one of the X's you would see in a batch triangle.
- **Nested Batch:** The homogeneous or Mimicker batch inside of the nesting batch. (Tiny white X inside of orange X.)

4. How to Fix It

The main thing to remember here was to look at the item as a single unit—a grouping. If at any point an item is needed or eaten currently in the grouping, make sure all items were

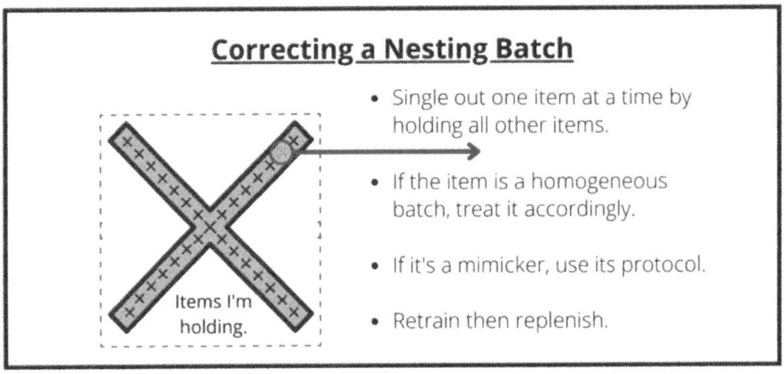
Correcting a Nesting Batch
Items I'm holding.
• Single out one item at a time by holding all other items.
• If the item is a homogeneous batch, treat it accordingly.
• If it's a mimicker, use its protocol.
• Retrain then replenish.

included. It had to be all or nothing every time a nested batch was included in the current batch. I would treat the current batch according to the type it was. With that being said, if I kept digging, I always found the connection. The connection always led to results.

5. How to Know If It Corrected

The nested batch was either a Mimicker or a homogeneous batch. The nested batch would be treated as a single unit of the nesting batch. The nesting batch could be any one of the three types. Both the nested batch and the nesting batch followed the same rules I shared already based on which type of batch they were.

If I previously appeared toxic and detoxing protocol was not working, taking supplements with the correct type of batch in mind corrected it. But remember, holding and taking all or nothing of the nested batch was key.

6. Key Takeaways

- The nested batch is either homogeneous or Mimicker.
    - Treat nested batch as a single unit.
    - Use the protocol for whatever type of batch it is.
- The nesting batch could be any of the three types.
    - Use the protocol for whatever type of batch it is.
    - Keep the Good Guys in with a manual DISH.
    - Fight Bad Guy while holding Bad Guy Byproduct or POOP.
- Watch for patterns in the supplements needed.
    - Groupings will reveal themselves.
    - Look for clues.

A nesting batch is a batch inside of a batch.

Personal Example

Sometimes pain or discomfort eventually just gets accepted without even realizing it. I always felt like I was babying my spleen. I wasn't even sure why I needed to. But I later came to find out, once I made the proper manual DISH, I was aware of the absence of pressure in my spleen area. Pressure I had felt for so long I didn't even realize it was there.

Time goes by and I started taking oxytocin supplements for a different problem. My daughter came to me and said every time I took oxytocin it made her spleen hurt. I did a Google search with just the words *spleen* and *oxytocin*. This information I'm about to share was revealed to me and I ran with it. I did the following batch on myself and it helped both of us. My DISH frequency helped her to sort the information she needed to sort too.

Example, lymphatic massage scenario.

As I mentioned before, I needed to manually make my DISH work. When I did, it revealed to me what a working DISH could do.

Bad Guy: Chlorobutanol. Chlorobutanol is a preservative used in medications, injections, oral sedatives, and topical anesthetics.[61]

> People also ask
>
> **What is Chlorobutanol used for?**
>
> It is a widely used preservative **in** various pharmaceutical solutions, especially injectables. Also, it is an active ingredient **in** certain oral sedatives and topical anesthetics. **Chlorobutanol** is a tertiary alcohol. **Chlorobutanol**, or chlorbutol, is an alcohol-based preservative with no surfactant activity [A32746].
>
> Chlorobutanol | C4H7Cl3O - PubChem
> pubchem.ncbi.nlm.nih.gov/compound/Chlorobutanol
>
> See all results for this question

Good Guy: Oxytocin. Oxytocin is a hormone the body needs.

Dilemma: Chlorobutanol mimics Oxytocin.[62]

> pubmed.ncbi.nlm.nih.gov › 4335551
>
> Responses of the isolated, perfused human spleen to ...
>
> The polypeptide **oxytocin** caused a slight vasodilatation in the human **spleen**, an effect almost exactly mimicked by the preservative chlorobutanol.8. Preliminary experiments suggest that...
>
> **Author:** A. B. Ayers, B. N. Davies, P. G. Withri... **Publish Year:** 1972

---

[61] PubChem. "Chlorobutanol." National Library of Medicine. Last accessed 28 March 2023. https://pubchem.ncbi.nlm.nih.gov/compound/Chlorobutanol.

[62] Ayers, A B, B. N. Davies, P. G. Withrington. "Responses of the Isolated, Perfused Human Spleen to Sympathetic Nerve Stimulation, Catecholamines and Polypeptides." National Library of Medicine. January 1972. https://pubmed.ncbi.nlm.nih.gov/4335551/.

My Perspective: For me, I was told I was *very toxic*. What do I mean? I was having a strong flare-up of inflammation. (My translation: Oxytocin—Bad Guy tug-of-war.) Taking supplements for detoxing my body was not working. I suspected I was toxic because I could not keep the oxytocin in. As I was trying to remove chlorobutanol, my oxytocin levels would drop with it.

Scenario: I decided to have a lymphatic massage while holding onto Good Guy (oxytocin). Massages are supposed to stimulate oxytocin AND I wanted to keep my roads open if it did *let the chemical go*. My DISH was working on its own more often than not at this point. I wanted to keep it that way. I did not want to overburden my body. By doing this, I reintroduced oxytocin into the system while manually doing the DISH's second job of sorting. Was the lymphatic massage necessary? I will never know. But I do believe holding oxytocin for my manual DISH was.

Afterwards: This did do the job I needed it to do. But because it did, I was exhausted for the next couple of days. Chlorobutanol is hard on the liver. I needed to let my body have time to process out all those chemicals. Meanwhile, I continued to maintain my manual DISH by holding oxytocin and chemical Byproduct.

Final Thoughts: This was not my first lymphatic massage, but it was my first one while holding oxytocin. It gave me profound results. Since this chlorobutanol was a Mimicker, twenty-four hours later, I needed to front load the supplement for oxytocin production.

Action Steps Summary

- The starting point is the same for each type of batch.
    - Start with holding item for forty-eight to fifty hours before I start taking it.
        - Easy step of programming & avoiding errant information.
        - Based on my reactions after this time period, I would know if I needed to do more.
        - This was usually enough.
    - Identify all known items for the batch, Good Guys and Bad Guys.
    - Hold them constantly or periodically, whichever was necessary.
- Start with the easiest type of batch, and if it didn't work, proceed to the next one or, as my body learned to communicate with itself, just ask what type of batch it was.
- The correcting process is different depending on the batch.
- Usually needed process of elimination.
    - Heterogeneous: Permission to Leave
        - Do a batch neutralizing session during this time.
        - Determine strongest or only meridian/organ being affected.
        - Determine what I need to continue to hold or take.
        - Repeat same batch twenty-four hours later—one session was for the organ and the other session was for its meridian.

    - Homogeneous: Get Kicked Out
        - Determine items for the batch.
        - Hold and consume Good Guy in small frequent doses over a long period of time.
        - Fight Bad Guy.
    - Mimicker: Seat Taken
        - Hold and avoid consuming for forty-eight to fifty hours.
        - Follow up with larger doses for a short period of time.
        - Hard on the body.
    - Nesting: A Batch Inside of a Batch
- Mimicker and nesting batches are the most difficult.
    - Hard to find what is being mimicked or grouped.
    - Time consuming searching for the connection.
    - Usually required holding for a minimum of nine months.
    - When the void is finally created to be refilled, there are challenges.
        - Temporarily highly sensitive to my environment.
        - Body will have a hard time functioning properly because of the temporary huge deficit of Good Guys while fighting the Bad Guy who has been poked.

Conclusion for Chapter 8

I know energy field manipulation is both *controversial* and *eccentric*, but the proof is in the pudding for me.

I know, it still boggles my mind too. I did all of this backwards. I would find what worked, then worked on figuring out why it was so. I have done my best to make sense of what I have noticed, what patterns I have found. I know I have found what works for me. I have found HOPE!

What if... this information could set someone else free too? How could I not share it?

How can I hold a Good Guy close to me and have the effect be greater than ingesting it?

For me to get my life back, the road was this way. It is not an easy road.

The instruction manual needed to be followed. If AFTER didn't work:

- Was I missing something from the batch?
- Was it a heterogeneous or homogeneous batch?
- Was the batch canceled?
- Was I able to identify a Mimicker?
- Which organ or meridian did I target?
- Was I trying to fight too much at once?
- Was it cycling?
- Was I systematically growing a batch?
- Was an allergen preventing me from progressing?
- Was I still circulating misinformation about a needed Good Guy I didn't know about yet?

AFTER is complex. It can be like following a flow chart to a computer program sometimes. The key takeaway from this approach was my body wanted to be well. The inflammation went away without drugs or essential oils or creams EVERY single time. All I had to do was narrow down the Good Guy(s) my body was rejecting and the type of batch they were in. I would then reprogram and end by placing item(s) on the outside of my body in order to maintain a manual DISH.

CHAPTER 9: CORRECTING THE MISSING INFORMATION

Reprogramming the brain

Opening Story: Just Breathe

After my hospital stay for my *panic attack* and before I had become so sensitive to everything again, I was just trying to survive day by day. This usually did not include a shower or combing my hair. If I did this, I wouldn't have enough energy to make sure my kids were fed and that the other must-dos were completed. Since it was Saturday, I thought maybe I could have enough strength to take a shower.

As I stood there testing the water flowing from the showerhead, I told myself, "I can do this." Removing my pajamas, which had become my standard uniform lately, I stepped into the stall. I leaned my hands up against the stall wall and just let the water pour over my head and down my back. It felt nice. I exhaled a sigh of relief followed by nothing. My lungs did not inhale as they naturally should have. They just did nothing. I tried inhaling on purpose. Nothing. What? Why can I not draw in a breath? After trying three times, I screamed in my head, *BREATHE*. I took in a breath, a deep breath. My, "Thank You God" was immediately followed up by my brain racing with the thought of why did my body not know to take a breath? I mused over the possibility of my body forgetting, and I wondered if this was happening with my other organs. Were they having a lack of communication too?

I kept taking the medication I was prescribed. But I couldn't shake this idea of the body forgetting, as crazy as it seemed. I sway tested the question, "Does my body know how to remove toxins?" The sway backwards to signify no was enough to cause my toes to come off the ground. What!? Why? This would explain a lot. I needed to put the why on the back burner for now and focus on a how.

I will share how in this chapter. But for now, I wanted to let you know that filling in this missing information enabled me to not be continually bedbound anymore. The before and after difference had me baffled. My body was obviously missing information. Important information. Information I would later realize was brought on by the misinformation causing nutritional deficiencies in my body. In particular, my vitamin Bs. I will elaborate on this in Chapter 11.

Overview

I believed I was open to this idea of retraining my brain because I had just finished using the book *The Gift of Dyslexia* by Ronald D. Davis and Eldon M. Braun. I saw before my eyes the transformation in my young teen. Not only did his reading and handwriting improve, but he no longer walked around with his head tilted. In this book, it talked about how some dyslexia was from disorientation. Correcting the disorientation corrected the head tilt even though we never targeted the head tilt specifically.

We hear of the benefits of relaxation and meditation for our health. We hear how we are supposed to focus on breathing during this time. This did not work for me either. The deep breathing seemed unproductive until I went through the process of reminding my body what the breathing was supposed to be doing. Yes, I know it sounds crazy and I can't explain exactly why it worked. I do know it caused a drastic improvement in my health I could not possibly explain in any other way.

The brain is an amazing thing, a baffling thing really. Sometimes just remembering a connection worked. It would help my body to understand how the different pieces of misinformation fit together. Other times I would need to tell my subconscious mind consciously and repeatedly what to do. Still other times, I needed to tell it how something was related to something else, or explain what two items were copying each other.

I will explain how I filled in my missing information in this chapter.

Topic 1: Laying the Groundwork

Correcting Missing Information

I needed to fill in the missing information from having a broken DISH. This process required being good at sway testing and developing a method of how to talk to my body. (How I sway tested is detailed in Appendix A.)

Talking to My Body

My mom was an amazing woman. She was also very smart. She was a "received an A in college calculus after being out of school for over a decade" type of smart. Unfortunately, she also had several strokes when she was only forty-two. She never recovered completely from them. It took her two years before she could eat, and another two before she could talk. She never regained use of her right side or had clear diction again.

BUT... she was totally mentally there. She had clarity of thought.

HOWEVER, something interesting happened. She could not subtract anymore. Period. We would ask her, "Mom, what is 2 + 3?" She would say, "Five." We would then immediately ask her, "Okay, then what is 5 – 3?" She could not tell us. No matter how many times we told her the answer, she could not remember it when it was subtraction. This would happen even when we would immediately ask her after the addition question.

So, before you dump the whole idea of sway testing, realize there is a little more technique involved than you may have previously thought.

Detox Organs

I had decided to see if I could retrain my body to detox. Stay with me here, I know it sounds crazy. I'm not talking about meditation, nor calmly taking in deep breaths; I'm talking about targeting different organs in the body and telling them—re-teaching them—what to do.

If I said, "Detox my body," nothing would happen. My body didn't understand what the phrase meant. In fact, it took almost four months of training before my body finally understood the command "detox the body." Through the process of systematically targeting one organ at a time, and telling it what to do, I could feel my body getting stronger. I could feel myself taking deeper breaths as I worked through each necessary organ. The deep breathing that didn't seem to do anything at all before.

The first day, I worked on this for over three hours! But persistence paid off. Eventually I came up with a script that I will share with you later.*

You may say, "I don't have three hours." Well, then you are healthier than I was. I was bedridden. This process took so long because, even though I'd just told my body what to do, it kept forgetting!

That very evening, and every day after, I had the strength to move about the house again. Occasionally, I did need to lie down and remind my body what to do. It usually took no more than ten minutes to get my body back on track. If I had known at this time my body was rejecting Good Guys, I may not have had to do this. I don't know. It's just a curious thought.

One day, after a couple of months training, I was busily focused on making supper, when suddenly the *script* entered my mind: "Have the liver, kidney, air sacs, skin, and nervous system act like any essential oil, remedy, or Bad Guy combination necessary in order to neutralize the toxins and release them from the body."*

Weird? It's like my body tried rebooting on its own. It was relearning! I didn't need to lie down to do it anymore!

Remind Body of Connections

I would also like to mention here when you have had low serotonin in the past, it is almost like you develop a feel for when it is normal or low, like a heart rate for other people. I don't need to test to see if my heart rate is up. I just know it is.

I got to the point where I could tell when my serotonin was low. I began to notice a pattern. I also noticed it would almost instantly switch back to normal. What caused this sudden switch? Mental connections.

Cartoon Mouse Analogy

For example, picture, if you will, a cartoon mouse having hundreds of cats chasing him down the alley. When he gets to the end of the alley, a big dog shows up standing where the mouse is heading. Suddenly, all the cats scatter and retreat. The mouse is overjoyed. He is liberated.

My brain was missing information. This mouse scenario is what it felt like for me. My mind was frantically sorting through countless cabinets of files trying to remember how something was connected to something else. Fatigue would set in.

It was like my brain needed to know the pathway, the connections, in order to allow the Bad Guy to know how to leave. Once the file was found, *boom*, everything was back to normal again. Kind of freaky.

The cats saw the dog and fled. The bogged-down feeling disappeared. Instantly.

When I would make a mental connection of how different objects or situations had certain things in common, it was like a click in the brain. The body now knew how to deal with what it was trying to remove from my body. My subconscious mind might not necessarily remember it later, but the conscious mind could remind it again. And again. As needed. I guess it was like trying to teach my kids to always put their shoes where they belong when they took them off. Hit and miss.

But the more frequently I told my body,

the more it became a hit.

This was my first jump toward better health. I was astonished and confused at it making such a big difference. It also made me realize I had a significant amount of reprogramming to do.

Topic 2: Missing Information Organ Detox

Keep in mind, if the information is not missing, this won't do anything. The body already knows what to do. However, the fact that it did work showed me my brain was missing the information.

Necessary background information

1. Before I attempted to do this, I needed to be well practiced with the sway test. See Appendix A.

2. I had spent the past ten days working on getting egg neutralized on all my meridians first. I do not know if this step is required. (Egg contains panthodic acid—see page 310) I only thought of this retraining concept after I had taken this step.

3. I talked to my body like a patient parent teaching a child how to learn something new. This would include detailed instructions and rechecking by asking if the body remembered what to do.

4. I know everything is connected and everything has unique nutrients and jobs associated with each organ. I also know I knew little about the specifics of it. However, this was like priming a pump to get the body going in the correct direction again. It was more about reminding the brain to communicate with the organs. The organs knew what to do; the brain just forgot to tell them to do it.

5. I had been using homeopathic remedies, essential oils, herbs, and the Emotion Code for about three years at this point. So, my body was familiar with what I was talking about when I would mention these things.

6. When it came to detoxing the lungs, it wouldn't work *until* I changed my wording to air sacs instead. I also needed

to mentally divide the lungs into small sections and do one section at a time.

7. I had with me what is called a MagBoy. It is two magnetic balls connected to each other with a casing around them. I wanted my energy to my brain to be the best it could, so I used this a few times before I began.

The wording is important. Do not say "detox."

Say "neutralize the toxins before they leave the body."

The Objective

The end goal of this training was to be able to prompt my body to reboot by summarizing what the body LEARNED during this session. I would say the following **target phrase**:

> *Have the liver, kidneys, gall bladder, air sacs, skin, and nervous system act like any essential oil, remedy, or Bad Guy combination necessary in order to neutralize the toxins and release them from the body, with and without emotions, memories, and other people's energy fields.*

This eventually transitioned over time. Baby steps of graduating through to simplifying the instructions.

1. "Do I remember the process to remove the toxins from the organs?"

a. If sway yes, say, "Do it."

b. If sway no, remind it of the target phrase.*

2. "Do I remember the process to detox?" (Then same as above for yes or no answers.)

a. Before this point, I actually had to train my body to know what the word *detox* meant. I did not attempt or think to do this, though, until about two weeks into the process. I only thought of it after I grew tired of repeating the phrase so much.

b. I treated it like a vocabulary card for detox that my body needed to learn. For example, "When I say detox the body, I mean have the liver, kidney..."

3. "Remember to detox."

4. Pinpoint particular items to detox when necessary. For example, when I unknowingly consumed MSG, my body was confused. I looked at the ingredients list and noticed it was there. I asked my body if it knew what it was. It did not. I ended up using the wording, "What I am trying to identify is MSG. It lacks any benefit to the body. Treat it like a toxin and remove it." It worked! The jitters went away instantly.

5. Eventually, my body no longer needed to be told. This took about six months. The first two weeks it was rather frequent reminders. It then gradually tapered to less and less frequently. The last leg, I think I went six weeks before I needed to remind it again.

Interestingly, over the years, I would know when something was going wrong because I would suddenly realize I was saying this same original script in my head subconsciously. It would be my signal to do something. My body was asking me for help.

How I Did It

1. I was alone in my room sitting on my bed with my back up against the wall. There were no distractions.

2. I ran the MagBoy over my head a few times.

3. I placed my hands on my core below the rib cage and asked my body if my blood was hurting. Remember, I used toddler speak to talk to my body. I don't think my body understood the concept of toxins yet.

4. I said, "These are toxins. We need to remove these toxins from the blood for the body to become well. Do I know how to do this?" (My sway was no.)

5. The conversation went a little like this. (I say *we* because I am referring to myself on two levels—my conscious and subconscious minds.)

- We need the brain to communicate with organs in the body that were designed to do this job. In order to communicate with these organs, we need the nervous system to have no toxins interfering. Do I know how to do this? (Sway is no.)
- We need these toxins to go into the blood so the body can remove them. Do I remember what toxins are? (Remind if necessary.)
- Do I know how to do this? (My sway is yes.) Do it.
- Am I doing it?
    - If yes, say keep doing it. (Pause.) Am I done for now?
    - If yes, focus on blood now.
    - If no, say keep doing it.
    - If no, is there too many toxins already in the blood?
    - If yes, say the organs in the body need to act like a filter to remove them.
- Start working on the target phrase* except focusing on one organ at a time.
    - Tell the specific organ to act like whatever essential oil or combinations of oils are

necessary to neutralize the toxins before they leave. (And proceed from there.)

- Frequently ask if toxic. Frequently ask if you know what to do. Frequently ask, "Can I do it?" Act on those responses as needed.

- If no, target the next organ.
- The order I did it in:

I needed to rotate through this group many times before adding more organs. Deep breaths and sighing are signs of progress.

- Nervous system
- Blood
- Gall bladder (needed to do this one twice)
- Liver
- Lungs—only worked if I said air sacs
- Kidneys
- Skin

If, when doing this, I could not take an adequate breath, it meant I needed to mentally divide the organ I was targeting into smaller pieces. For example, at one point I needed to break the right area of the lung into twelve parts. Target air sacs in part one only. Target air sacs in part two only, etc. Whenever I needed to do this, once I was done, I would start over at the beginning to *make more room for toxins to leave*.

Keep in mind, this was a slow process. I have touched on the highlights to give you an idea of what I am talking about. It took me three hours.

Over the next several days, I continually checked to see if my body was still *doing it*. I also would remind it as necessary to keep doing it. It took a significant amount of reminding for the first month. It then tapered off into gradually longer gaps.

Gradually, the breaths became deeper and bigger.

Doing this process, my body voluntarily took deeper breaths without needing to focus on the idea of taking a deeper breath.

Another Process I Also Needed to Teach

"When there is no food for the body to make serotonin, automatically go to the fat stores and convert (key word) the fat to energy (key word) so the body can make serotonin."

Once trained, I needed to remind my body a few times after each meal to return to food stores of fat and to check back regularly every five minutes to see if there is food to utilize. Occasionally, I would get the result of fat too toxic to use. By knowing this, I would know I needed to work on something.

Topic 3: Reprogram Other Information

Knowing When There Is Missing Information

Short answer: Sway test and ask myself, "Am I missing information?" Act on the answer.

Long answer: Missing information is less frequent. It seemed to correct with the misinformation being corrected. Remember the tight connection. The misinformation caused the Good Guy deficiency, which in turn caused missing information. Sometimes just correcting the misinformation is enough for the missing information to correct. I do not have this down to an art yet. (Most reprogramming was needed for

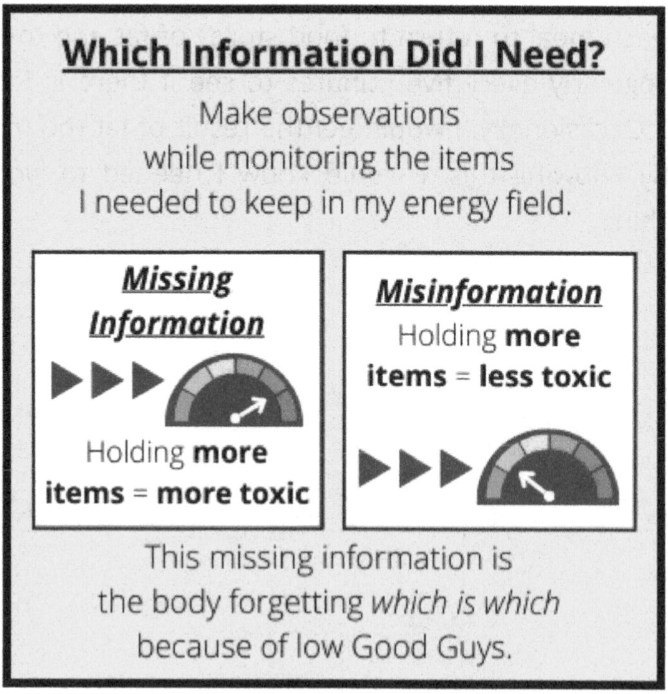

Which Information Did I Need?
Make observations
while monitoring the items
I needed to keep in my energy field.
Missing Information
Holding more items = more toxic
Misinformation
Holding more items = less toxic
This missing information is
the body forgetting which is which
because of low Good Guys.

misinformation.) The only way I knew I was needing to reprogram missing information was by monitoring the items I needed to keep in my energy field. If the more items I held, the more toxic I became, it was a sign of missing information. If the more items I held, the less toxic I became, it was a sign of misinformation. This missing information is the body forgetting which is which.

For example, I did not know, and therefore could not reprogram, the missing information about a nutrient I needed for my intestines. Gabatone. My doctor asked me if I had ever taken it before. No. He asked if I thought it was what I needed. I had never heard of it, nor did I know what it was. My body did not make any connection to the information. There was not a sway yes or no. It literally had no idea what it was. The doctor went and retrieved it from the other room, and the second he crossed the threshold to return to the room I was in, I swayed so far forward it almost knocked me out of my chair. I proceeded to yawn big and frequently, almost having a difficult chance to recatch my breath in between the multiple yawns.

Many a time while thinking about what I would need to hold or take for the day, there would be a change in my breathing pattern. If that happened, I would immediately ask myself if this was missing information. If yes, whatever the mental connection was, I would repeat it periodically for about ten minutes, sometimes twenty minutes. After doing this, most times I would not need to hold or take the item.

How to Reprogram the Missing Information

1. ***Look for what is missing.***

- A repeated incomplete batch could indicate a mental connection was missing.
    - This could even be a scent of something.
    - What was it made of?
    - How was it connected to each item already in the batch?
- Knowing there is a connection, but not what it is.
    - Problem item: For example, tainted estrogen—an area of my body where I was having trouble having enough good estrogen.
    - Solution item: A similar essential oil or homeopathic remedy:
        - Hold it in my energy field.
        - Tell my body to recognize it, correct it, and allow the tainted stuff similar to it to leave—took twenty minutes.
        - Hold for the next forty-eight hours, periodically remind myself.
- Consider the different ways batches are made and look for connections.
    - Exposure
    - Proximity
    - Resemblance
- Sometimes all the items in a batch are known, but how they are connected is the missing piece.
    - Treat it like a mind game.
    - Find how they are connected by researching.
        - Research item.
        - Research part of body being affected.

2. Reprogramming the information.

Similar to the example I gave to the organ detox method, I would talk to my body and tell it the information it needed. During this time, I would continually ask if it remembered, or if I was winning, or the like. While doing this, I used to bob my head forward with frequent yeses. I thought this was insignificant and not even worth mentioning in the book until my recent doctor's appointment. He shared with me how to, as he would say, defrag my brain. This head bobbing forward was a way of resetting the nervous system. Who knew!? I didn't. I was just doing what worked and not knowing why.

Hence, while I did this head bob, I would continually tell myself the information I needed to know. It usually took ten minutes and then reminders periodically every couple of hours for a day or two.

3. Knowing when the missing information is found.

For a picture, it would look like a child walking down the sidewalk and then suddenly deciding to do a couple of skips out of joy of excess energy. There will be a skip, a change of some kind. I call this a change in my breathing pattern. It could be a cough, yawn, shortness of breath, shallow breathing, sneeze, one deep inhale, gasping for air, hiccups, or a combination.

If the missing information was found, I wouldn't stop there. I'd do a mental check of what possible nutrients may be lacking to cause it. I'd replenish those nutrients to avoid the information from getting lost again.

The disconnects needed to be fixed and prevented.

Personal Examples

Back during the beginning of my decision to follow my own path, I recall a trip I had taken to the local health food store. I was searching for a particular item. It was supposed to help with chicken pox. It was out of stock. The cashier assisting me at the time mentioned maybe trying a different product because it was for herpes. He thought it might work since they were in the same family of virus. The second he said the last sentence, it was like my body got taller and a deep breath came rushing in. It caught me off guard. It was the first time I experienced it for something other than detoxing my organs and reminding them how to work. Over the following years, I started noticing I would experience the change in breathing pattern or the sudden burst of energy when a mental connection was finally made. Do I understand it? No. Did it happen? For me, every time.

Action Steps Summary

- I reprogrammed my detox organs.
- I would continually recheck and remind my body what it should be doing.
- I would observe what situation was taking place while working on batches.
    - If holding more items made me more toxic, I was missing information.
    - Search for the missing information.
        - ✓ Look for patterns in supplements or remedies prescribed.
        - ✓ It's difficult because I didn't know what I was missing until it was found.

- Correct missing information.
    - Reprogram the nervous system with the required information.
    - Use any technique recommended to facilitate this.
    - Replenish nutrients causing the missing information.
    - Keep those nutrients manually in my DISH.

Conclusion for Chapter 9

Yes, this may seem like a guessing game. However, knowing where to look based on how batches are made enabled the guessing to be more focused. The amazing part is, regardless of how many times I did this process, when I found the missing information, I would always have a change in my breathing pattern. After which I was able to complete the batch and move on.

After the organ detox protocol, most of my time was spent manually doing batches to correct misinformation and prevent loss of the Good Guys. Keeping the Good Guys in was crucial to prevent missing information from happening again. But because the information was missing, it did need to be reinserted again. This method was how I did the process.

At this point you are probably thinking it sounded pretty complicated. I know. It was frustrating. It was frustrating continually needing to search for connections. It was hard to search for something when I didn't know what I was searching for.

How did I know for certain it was working? My body was getting stronger. It was fighting problems I had encountered in my distant past. It made sense of them still being there. If the body was too weak to fight it, why on earth would the Bad Guy leave of its own accord? It wouldn't. With that being said, here is where it is like Pandora's box. The body was not removing the Bad Guys for a reason. But my body wanted to be well. The minute it saw an opportunity, it would try. This was not always safe, easy, or pretty as I will get into in the next chapter.

Section 4

Magnitude of DISH

CHAPTER 10: EASIER SAID THAN DONE

The concept is easy; implementing it is difficult.

Opening Story: My Routine to Leave the House

The key here was my body would be exposed to several different Bad Guys whenever I changed my environment. If my body wasn't sorting those Bad Guys, I needed to be altering the shield manually. I would want to start off with at least maintaining my shield before I left my house. It would begin with educated guesses based on patterns, followed up with sway testing.

What follows is a description of a typical day for me to leave the house. I still do this, but to a significantly lesser degree.

1. I would need to sway test and determine what main item(s) I would need for the artificial coating for the day. I would soak in the tub with them for ten minutes to an hour.[63]

2. After getting out of the tub, I would need to strategically reapply the items I needed on specific areas of my body to keep the Good Guy(s) in so I could continue to fight the Bad Guy(s). I was now at my baseline.

3. I had a select amount of standard Good Guys I always seemed to need when I left the house. I just kept a small

[63] A handful of times, this maxed out at four hours. But that would be one of those days or nights I wasn't going anywhere. In these situations, something was usually missing from the batch.

sample of each in my purse and never took them out. This way, I didn't need to think about it.

4. I would need to add in any other items my sway test was telling me I needed to take with me. Sometimes stuffed in my pockets, socks, or bra and other times added to my purse.

5. Since I needed to be the strongest energy field, I would sit on a magnetic chair pad whenever I drove. The first year of finally being able to drive, I also had a magnetic pad on my front. I looked like a sandwich. I had to accept the possibility of people thinking I'm weird. After three years of not being able to even be a passenger in a car without feeling incredibly nauseous, I was just glad I could take my kids to their activities and stay to watch.

6. I had to be selfish. No matter what, if I was unable to do the tub soaking during the spleen meridian clock, nine to eleven a.m., I would have to be home to soak for the small intestine meridian clock, one to three p.m. This was the case for me because these were the areas I needed to be targeting.

7. I needed to be mindful of my environment, because if challenges came up later in the day, it could be because of something I was exposed to during my time-out. It could be I just needed a quick release from it or it may have triggered the next item my body felt it could fight now.

8. That being said, it was easier to just stay home as much as I could. This is less frequently the case now. I am to the point now where I don't even need my magnetic pad anymore when driving.

I improved because I continually did the work. I kept doing what worked until I could find out why it worked. Figuring out that my body needed to keep L-Aspartic Acid and oxytocin in was incredibly significant in reducing the effort it took to be able to leave the house. Realizing the chlorinated hydrocarbon and pesticide connection enabled me to start exercising again.

Overview

The best way to describe what is going on is to look at it like a video game. The first levels are easy, but each level becomes more difficult whether it be because of sheer quantity or aggressiveness of the enemy. I don't know if levels can be skipped to jump to killing the mother ship, so to speak. The body may need to make itself stronger first by passing all the other levels. Removing all other Bad Guys so all my focus can be directed at only the mother ship. Does that make sense?

Once the mother ship was there to fight, I would need to focus on only it. This was when all supplements must stop except for the ones specifically needed to target destroying the mother ship.

Now, when I start to shoot this Bad Guy, I won't get very far shooting wildly everywhere on the screen. My best bet was constant repeated direct hits. This is how I did that. Depending on the type of Bad Guy, Mimickers were usually the most difficult. It was like flushing out a water system—the Bad Guy needed to be removed before the Good Guy could be inserted. If it flowed both ways, so to speak, it would just be jumbled. No progress.

Sometimes finding the Bad Guy is easy; other times not so much. But the key here is the Bad Guy may never be known sometimes. It helps to know it so I can determine the batch it is in, but it isn't necessary. The main culprit we are looking for is the Good Guy who isn't sticking around. Holding it makes it stay.

For an easy example, in the case of Camp Lejeune water contamination, strontium-90 was in the water—Bad Guy. Obvious Good Guy was strontium, a mineral the body needs for many functions such as bone growth. Easy enough. But not so easy.

- **Exposure:** Lead from X-ray vests
- **Proximity:** Thyroid (iodine) targeted by radiation
- **Resemblance:** Cobalt-60 is radiation as well

For a difficult example, again with Camp Lejeune water problems, let's look at vinyl chloride. Vinyl chloride is a type of plastic. Plastic is a polymer.[64] Collagen is a polymer too.[65] According to Wikipedia, collagen makes up about twenty-five to thirty-five percent of the whole-body protein content. [66]

- **Exposure:** Plastic used everywhere
- **Proximity:** Many parts of the body including lungs and brain
- **Resemblance:** Polyester

---

[64] RSPAdmin. "Polymer vs Plastic." RSP Inc. Manufacturing Partner. 28 October 2019. https://www.rspinc.com/blog/plastic-injection-molding/polymer-vs-plastic/.

[65] Umber Cheema, Michael Ananta, and Vivek Mudera. "Collagen: Applications of a Natural Polymer in Regenerative Medicine." IntecOpen. 29 August 2011. https://www.intechopen.com/chapters/19026.

[66] Wikipedia. "Collagen." Wikipedia. Last edited 15 March 2023. https://en.wikipedia.org/wiki/Collagen.

For an amazingly difficult example (but it still followed the rules), we have a known contaminant of chlorinated hydrocarbons—insecticide. Bad Guy. Through many weeks of studying the patterns I knew, I believed this was what I was working on. I also kept coming up with lipids as being a factor. I don't even know how I remembered this name from biology class, but there it was. I finally decided to try to understand what lipids did in the body, so I looked the word up on Google. Guess what popped up? Lipids are hydrocarbons! There was my Good Guy.

- **Exposure:** On all non-organic food
- **Proximity:** Cells, organs, and tissues (ugh!)
- **Resemblance:**
  - ✓ **Good Guy:** Phosphorus
  - ✓ **Bad Guy(s):** Pharmaceuticals, plastics, and solvents[67]

> Chlorinated hydrocarbons are chemical compounds of chlorine, hydrogen, and carbon atoms only. Many of them form the building blocks of other chemical products such as pharmaceuticals, plastics, and solvents.
>
> www.epa.gov/eg/chlorine-and-chlorinated-hydrocarbon-manufacturing-industry
>
> Chlorine and Chlorinated Hydrocarbon Manufacturing Industry

[67] EPA—United States Environmental Protection Agency. "Chlorine and Chlorinated Hydrocarbon Manufacturing Industry." EPA Gov. Last updated 24 April 2020. https://www.epa.gov/eg/chlorine-and-chlorinated-hydrocarbon-manufacturing-industry.

Topic 1: Finding the Bad Guy

Sometimes it may feel like looking for a needle in a haystack. This venture may seem impossible, but it was much more doable if I had a magnet. Studying patterns for DISH was my magnet—my secret weapon, so to speak. It may not be easy, but you need to realize the jump I was making wasn't from easy to easier. The attempt I was undergoing was from not doable to possible.

In order to understand this invisible enemy I was dealing with, I needed to study batches. Batches are where the Bad Guys always hung out. Remember, there are three ways to describe a batch: how it's made, the status, and what type. Knowing this made it easier to know what to do. Why? Because we need to single out the Bad Guy to fight it. (Isolate the frequency to cancel the frequency.) Remember, this Bad Guy could be one thing or a group of things. Once this Bad Guy was singled out and neutralized, it needed to be repeated with all the other Bad Guys in his gang.

Sometimes this needed assistance and sometimes it didn't. Most of the time for me, when two big Bad Guys have been neutralized by themselves, they needed help when they were put together even though they both were already neutralized. The two of them together were a different frequency. This made them, as a team, a whole new problem.

This may seem overwhelming, but the body is an incredible thing. It does this all without a hitch when the DISH is functioning properly. Please don't feel overwhelmed. It took me ten years to figure out what I am shoving down your throat as fast as you can read this book.

Three Possible Methods

Three possible methods to find the Bad Guy.

1. I am told by a homeopath, naturopath, or doctor who the Bad Guy is.

2. I hear about it on the news or from Google searches.

3. I have a list of common environmental exposures I was exposed to.

If Those Methods Didn't Work

I still had one more way to try to find the Bad Guy. It was a four-step process, sway testing everything I did along the way.

1. Hold the Good Guys. This batch will get large, but remember, I only need a trace amount. Even if it is up to fifty items, it could fit in a small Ziploc baggie.

2. Damage will be occurring until the DISH is equalized.
  - **a.** Essential oils to reduce damage.
  - **b.** Magnets to aid in quicker healing.

3. Study my medical history and life.
  - **a.** List significant events or illnesses.
  - **b.** Write out the exposure batches that may have occurred during this time.
  - **c.** Search for resemblance batches of similarities and common ground items.

4. Research the result I find.
  - **a.** Look for a missing piece to a resemblance batch.
  - **b.** Look for a Bad Guy similar to a Good Guy.
  - **c.** The fewer key words in Google search, the better.
    - **i.** Area of body being affected and item

ii. Potential Bad Guy and current Good Guy deficiency
iii. Organs being affected and Good Guys needed for them

Narrowing Down the Search

There are two ways the misinformation may have occurred.

1. A Bad Guy was/is mimicking a Good Guy.
2. A Good Guy was mixed with a Bad Guy.

Either way, the key was the Good Guy. Let the Good Guy stay around so it can do its job. Having a functioning DISH allowed this to happen. Holding the correct Good Guy allowed the DISH to function properly when it could not automatically.

Anything Is Game

A frequency is a frequency. Everything has energy so everything has frequency. It means it could be absolutely anything. I've had it be an item from the environment, an emotion, a sound, a color, or a combination of things. But when the match is found, it always kicks in and I always end up better off than I was.

It would be nice if there was a database for this. Someday maybe there will be. Meanwhile, sometimes it takes a long time to find the answer. It took me nine months to figure out the connection between collagen and plastic. I think it was because they were both polymers. It took me two years to figure out the pesticide and lipid connection. I know. Sad numbers. I won't lie. It is very frustrating at times. I press on because the knowledge of knowing it will work every single time (so far). It's just finding what other people probably already know, but they just don't know the significance of what they know yet.

Topic 2: Surviving the Battle

The number one problem is it is uncharted territory. Who knows what lies around the next bend, so to speak. For example, if you hang around health stores a lot, we hear about chelating metal. Done it. Tried it. Poor results. I was putting in the work but nothing seemed to change. But when I did DISH, it did. The die-off that ensued was incredible.

If this was the equivalent of poking the bear, at least I could try to run away from it. However, it was more like trap doors. Trap doors in uncharted territory. Walking along and not seeing the trip wire. The ground underneath me suddenly giving out.

Trap Doors

It wasn't until years later that I realized what I was doing was sort of like an all-or-nothing ordeal. I have heard of people talking about detoxing slowly or quickly and speeding up the process or slowing down the process. Well, the problem with what I figured out was that adjusting the speed was not an option. When the combination was figured out, it was more like a trap door opening up. The only thing at this point was to protect the body the best I could. The best way to do that was to get as close a match as possible.

On the good side, learning to hold proximity Good Guys during this time helped incredibly. I could continue to get better.

On the bad side, the healthier I got, the more my body fought. When I got these bad guys to start moving, it got pretty tough on the organs. Remember the trap door scenario I was talking about? Well, sometimes a trap door released a long-overdue flood. If this flood was unwanted metals in the body, there seemed to be almost a type of friction damage going on from the speed of it leaving. (Metals are tiny crystals. Crystals can cut.) I never thought this was possible. I was always told I needed to push pretty hard to get those metals out. Well, maybe not. I just needed to find the combination to open the trap door. Kaboom!

Dump vs. Drop

A dump is when there is a surge of toxins because the body now has permission to get rid of the Bad Guy. A dump would also need to be followed up by periodically touching the batch triggered by it. A drop is a done deal. It is over. No need to periodically touch the batch. It is just necessary to hold the Good Guy Kingpin (rod).

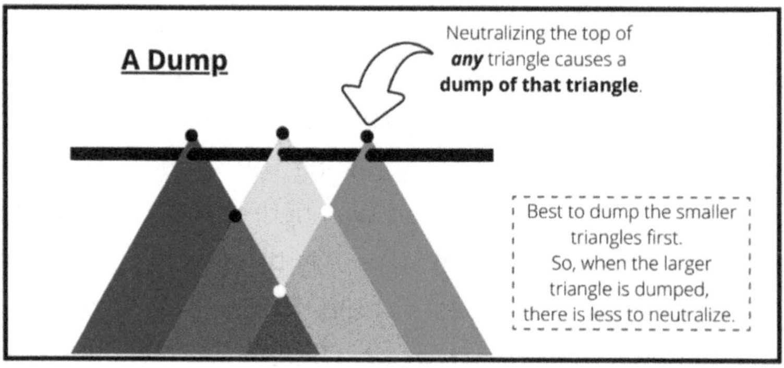

A Dump
Neutralizing the top of any triangle causes a dump of that triangle.
Best to dump the smaller triangles first. So, when the larger triangle is dumped, there is less to neutralize.

A drop always involves a Kingpin. It holds on to more than one batch. It is a dumping of multiple batches. At this point, the key is to keep the lymphatic system open and to keep pulling out the *debris* (Byproduct & POOP) building up very quickly in the body. Taking any nutritional supplements to speed this up would be harmful to me. Only binders would be beneficial. Using the bike analogy again, we are pedaling as fast as we can. We don't want the chain to get knocked off (sorting to stop).

This drop is able to occur because the reprogramming has been done. I only needed to hold what current supplements I was taking at this time for prevention purposes. Sometimes it also included the Good Guys for the organ I was targeting. I wanted to avoid creating a new batch because of proximity.

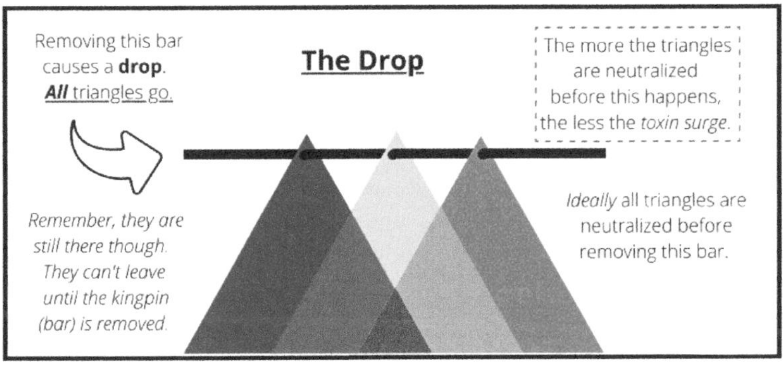

The goal is to only have the drop occur after the batches involved in the drop have had everything in them canceled. The less is canceled, the larger the toxicity load of processing out what gets activated. One time I inadvertently triggered a drop without realizing I was building up to it. I didn't realize glycine was mimicking aspirin. The amazing thing was, even if I didn't really know why I needed to do something, by doing it, my body would run with the opportunity to be well.

Controlling the Dumps and Drops

The only way to control this was to try to do as many dumps as possible before removing the Kingpin. The dumping is controlled by what triangle top I focused on. Ideally, I would want all the triangles to be neutralized. It somehow created fewer toxins that way. Less damage. Canceled is canceled.

Regardless, when a dump or a drop has occurred, this is when I usually needed to stop boosting my body's strength (stop most supplements) and focus on binders to protect my body. During this processing time, the body (especially the detox organs) were at risk of being mixed.

For example, when my body was finally able to release a Bad Guy in my small intestines, my kidneys went into overdrive, so to speak. My kidneys worked fine, but were getting overburdened. There was a tipping point when my kidneys were getting worked too hard processing. I knew this because supplements to heal my kidneys started showing up on my sway tests.

Proceed with Caution

Obviously, when these Bad Guys have built up in my body over a long period of time, there ends up being a lot of them. So... when the trap door is opened, watch out.

Die-Off

It was very hard on my kidneys. Could friction alone possibly cause problems, let alone my body trying to process it out? I have enclosed a picture to demonstrate. I know a before and after picture would be more ideal, but I wasn't expecting it to happen. I'm asking you to believe me when I say both legs and feet (minus the black sores) looked the same before I did my procedure. After I did my procedure, the following morning my leg and foot were swollen. (I was targeting my right kidney.) Also, true to the pattern, coughing started up 48 hours later. Based on what I needed to do to help it to go away, it was die-off from what I did.

BTW: Those sores were on many places on my body for years. What I share in this book is what finally made them go away.

Are you curious to know the way I finally was able to remove those black sores from my body? After having them for years and using both topical and oral medications during that time, I decided to test my new ideas. Instead of taking these liver supplements orally, I placed them in a tiny jar and carried it around with me all the time. I continued to treat the sores topically as well. Eventually, what appeared to be a

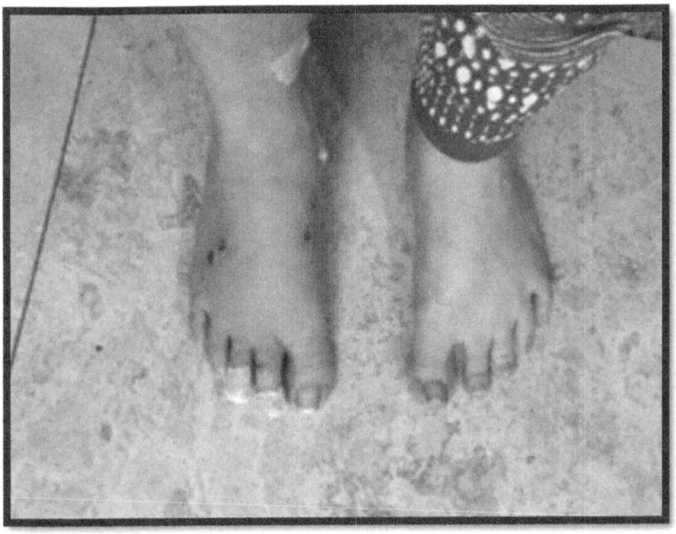

lymphatic parasite showed up next to the largest black hole (size of a U.S. quarter). This area next to the hole bled a little when the object left. This hole, and the other smaller ones, went away. It took about four months. Four months was nothing considering I had been dealing with them for years.

Voids

When reprogramming happens, regardless of what type of batch it is, there has to be a change in command, so to speak. The Bad Guy has to leave before the Good Guy can take his place. Sometimes it isn't quick. Picture a hose. I can't have water going in and out at the same time. I had to wait until the out process was completed first.

- The hole left behind depended on what the Bad Guy created.
- How and when to refill it depended on the type of batch it was.

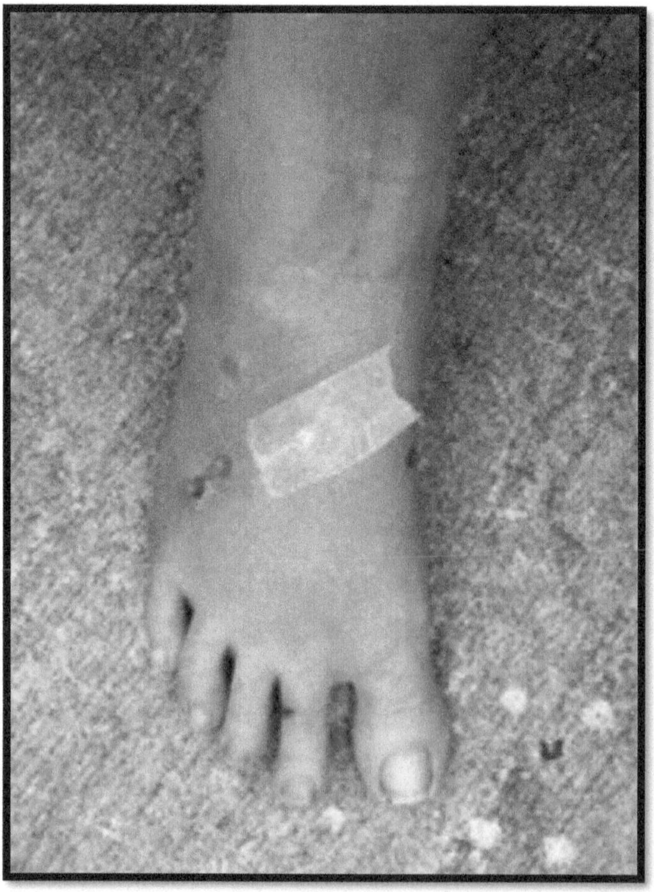

Topic 3: Knowing I'm Making Progress

It's a long game with small checkpoints.

Consequences of Drops

When a Kingpin is found, holding it will cause the trap door to open. Everything has an exit. We have a drop. I could tell I was approaching a Kingpin when I needed to be holding several items and to avoid taking any supplements. Even detox supplements at this point would cause swelling and my body wanting to power down to protect itself from rejecting the mimicked nutrient too fast. Once this nutrient was discovered and held, the trap door would go and I would no longer need to hold any of the items. I would also be able to slowly start adding supplements back into my regimen to gradually start growing the next batch.

Remember my L-Aspartic Acid example? I was needing to hold onto over thirty different items at one point. I couldn't figure out who the Mimicker was. When I narrowed it down to what was being mimicked, L-Aspartic Acid, holding it caused the drop. I immediately no longer needed to hold all those items. The first four days after a drop are usually exhausting, but then it is always followed up by a jump in my overall health. Everything in the batch is now a nonissue. They are removed. I no longer needed to hold any of those items, nor touch them purposefully again.

Relief Shows Up

Sometimes when I have been sick for a long time, for a really long time, I almost forget what some of my symptoms are. I learn to live with them. They are the normal, so I don't think to mention it. In fact, for me, I even learned to completely shut it out at one point without even realizing it.

When working on a batch, I came across the need for vanadium. So, step one, I taped it on my spleen area not thinking anything of it. Two hours later, I was suddenly aware of the absence of dull pain. I felt like my body took a deep sigh of relief. I don't know how else to describe it.

This also happened with cysteine and my kidneys. My body felt a sigh of relief and I was able to be more active.

One evening, my liver had been really sore all day. Unable to be a contributing member of society type of sore. I was missing something. I looked at the homeopathic remedies I had been needing to hold and I looked at the list of supplements I had been needing to take and chose glutathione. Why?

I had recently found out glutathione is used in some vaccinations. The virus remedy I was holding was one such vaccination. I only recently learned of this information because of the TV show playing in my doctor's office at my last appointment. Talk about timing.

This time, maybe it was because I was acutely aware of it, or because it was the only item left in the batch, but within twenty minutes the pain was gone! Was I glad? Yes. But I couldn't believe I hadn't thought of it earlier in the day. It did take about six hours, though, before the big sigh of relief came. For example, if this was like the stomach flu, the twenty-minute marker would be when I finally stopped throwing up. The six-hour marker was when I felt human again and was back to being able to converse and sit on the couch.

Batches Become Smaller with Bigger Players

In the beginning of this process, it was mostly heterogeneous batches. However, they were very large batches in the batch neutralizing sessions. It was better to have a minor something I didn't need than to not have what I needed. An incomplete batch, regardless of how big it was, would cancel when I ate or drank something. I would have to start over.

However, as the batches became smaller, they rarely contained minor allergens and *insignificant items*. They would be centered around the more intimidating Bad Guys.

Personal Examples

Narrowing Down the Culprit

I am still trying to work on a system to make this easier. I am still looking for more obvious patterns. But for now, it is so much easier looking back and noticing the pattern was there all along. But the more I looked back, the more I saw the patterns appearing ahead. This enabled me to start tweaking it. To start really nailing down the little differences that made a big difference. Sometimes I do not know what caused the trap door to drop until after it had happened. Sometimes I thought I was doing a homogeneous batch and got surprised by a Mimicker. Only recently did I realize I was working on a Mimicker who was also located in a homogeneous batch. (I explained this in Chapter 8.)

Yes, it gets complicated. But so far, so good. Figuring out what type of batch it is and doing the required steps has worked. It has stopped pain, inflammation, candida overgrowth, and the need for so many supplements.

Sometimes It's Complicated

This is not meant for medical advice. This is just an example of how complicated it can be. I wouldn't wish this on anyone. I was targeting methylmercury with mumps. The items I used in the batch were based on studying the three ways batches are formed. This was an alternating batch.

1. I held Super Enzyme in my energy field for two complete meridian clock cycles. So, fifty hours is a safe bet, generally speaking.

- **a.** This separated the Super Enzyme from the methylmercury w/mumps.
- **b.** It was very important NOT to take this supplement during the time that the body was working on identifying it.
- **c.** My body now recognized what was methylmercury w/mumps and what was Super Enzymes.

2. When doing this, the Super Enzyme was directly taped on the surface of my skin where the large intestines are located for one complete large intestine (LI) meridian clock (five to seven a.m.) and the next time cycle on a LI meridian point. (The order this is done in doesn't seem to matter.) Even though the meridian clock has only two-hour segments, I seemed to need three hours, thirty minutes on each side of the window.

3. The first four days (note I am targeting methylmercury w/mumps individually and in combination):

- **a.** During the five to seven a.m. window (Target: methylmercury w/mumps):
    - **i.** Take one Super Enzyme and wait thirty minutes.
    - **ii.** Take half a Super Enzyme caplet, wait ten minutes.
    - **iii.** Take another half caplet, wait for ten more minutes.
    - **iv.** Warning: If I move from my spot, drink anything, or eat anything, I lose. I won't be strong enough to fight it. I do not want my energy fields changing. It will be like adding back in all the other energy fields before I had a chance to correct the target.
        1. Not only do I lose, but I also have to go back to the beginning.
        2. If I mess up this step, even if I am on day three, I have to start the entire four-day cycle all over.
    - **v.** Drink some lymphonest.
- **b.** During the one to three p.m. small intestine meridian window (Target: methylmercury):
    - **i.** Plan to stay in one place, preferably alone for twenty to twenty-five minutes.
    - **ii.** Take L-Methionine, Taurine, Cataplex C, Valine, Serine, Dopa Mucuna, and wait twenty minutes.
    - **iii.** Drink some lymphonest.

c. Throughout the day (Target: mumps):
    i. Hold lymphonest constantly in my energy field and drink as needed.
    ii. Vivi virox as needed.

4. Rested two days to allow toxins to process out.
    a. I constantly tested to make sure toxins were not being held back by a missing nutrient.
    b. If it is, it may mean there is another factor involved. For me it was egg and aluminum.
        i. Omega
        ii. Licking an aluminum beater (believe it or not)

5. Next four days (because of benzene poisoning of water):
    a. Whatever batch I did, I always had to repeat it with benzene.
    b. To mimic benzene, I used Cataplex C (½, ¼, ¼) and Detoxosode (I was out of TMG).
    c. I took these two supplements with the Super Enzymes batch.
    d. Everything else was done the same as before for the rest of the day.

6. The third four days:
    a. Here is the tricky part—there is always one last chain link to allow the release to happen.

   b. This is where understanding how groupings are made is helpful.
   c. For me it was methylmercury w/Lortab mimicking or grouped with glutathione.
      i. I held glutathione constantly to "make" methylmercury w/Lortab stay on the front lines.
      ii. Detoxosode.
      iii. Lymphonest.
7. Aftermath
   a. Slowly start adding back in the supplements.
   b. Every supplement I added allowed me to grow the size of the batch I was fighting.
   c. Try to control the die-off through oils and soaking and whatnot.
   d. For some reason, the usual, like clay and Modifilan, would not work.
   e. Potassium citrate seemed to help the most.
      i. Sometimes only needing to hold it.
      ii. Sometimes needing to take it with L-Citrulline.
   f. I limited my diet (raw food only) during the aftermath to allow toxins to leave easier. I didn't want my body getting distracted with digesting.

Action Steps Summary

I truly believe my body wanted to be well. I am forcing a broken piece of this body to work. Since I didn't know what I was looking for, I didn't know what I would find. I also didn't realize how backed up or how evil of a Bad Guy(s) was behind the blockage until they revealed themselves.

- Bad Guys can be really bad.
  - Get outside help.
  - Keep searching for connections.
  - Protect myself by learning what I can about what I was up against as soon as I knew what it was.
  - Neutralize as many smaller triangles (batches) as possible before targeting larger triangles or Kingpins.
- Get out of the way to let the bad stuff leave.
  - Hold Byproduct or POOP whenever possible for the Bad Guy(s).
  - Hold any proximate Good Guy(s) necessary to allow progress.
  - Keep an arsenal of ways to detox my body in different situations.
- Don't grow weary in doing good.
  - Doubt is gone—my invisible illness has been revealed.
  - Helplessness is gone—I can do something about my health.
  - Don't have to wait to be done to feel better.

Conclusion for Chapter 10

Why would anyone want to go through all this trouble? Please remember, it wasn't like I had a choice. The life I once lived was gone. I wanted it back. There was no way up and out of the situation I was in. I felt like I was playing Russian roulette whenever I ate anything. Who knew what would happen. There was no logical explanation for the problems I was having. Regardless, I could not leave my home, nor function at home on even a slightly normal basis. I could not eat without foam rising in my throat making it hard to breathe. (One of the symptoms my mom used to have as well, with no answers.) Where did it get her? Strokes! Strokes at the age I was currently at.

Though it was a hassle, I realized by doing the things in this book, I was able to slowly get my life back. I was able to eat again. I was able to be inside around electricity again. I was even able to be in front of a computer again. I was able to drive places. Go into stores. Take my daughter shopping. So many daily life privileges that can be easily taken for granted.

I think back to when I first went to a homeopath. She had looked at me after running some tests. I could never forget the look on her face.

She said, “You have been sick for a long time.”

My husband answered, “Yeah, for about a year.”

She replied, “No, she has been sick for a very long time.”

She looked directly at me and said, “For over a decade.”

I suppressed my cry of relief and freedom. Somebody finally believed me.

At the time, she said it would take a year. A year? It seemed so long. But if the choice was a year or forever, I guess I’ll take the year. She was able to get me better in nine months. However, at this plateau I had reached, I knew I could not stay. My diet was incredibly limited. There was no way I could get the right quantity of Good Guys to be able to stay at this plateau.

If I knew then what I know now, I think the path would have been much shorter. Maybe I would have been totally better with what she did if I knew my body wasn't sorting. I may never know.

Yes, I am still doing this manual sorting. When I do, my life is almost normal. I am not waiting around for something outside of my control to eventually show up to make me better. I can immediately tell now when my body stops sorting. Manually doing the sorting gets my body back online. Even though there are tough days or tough times of the day, they are getting fewer and farther apart. It was advantageous to know the patterns to make those times, though not always avoidable, at least somewhat predictable.

As I look back now, my homeopath was correct. I had been sick for a long time, a very long time. Now I know why, and it wasn't just in my head.

"Life can only be understood backwards, but it must be lived forwards." —Søren Kierkegaard

---

CHAPTER 11: HIDING IN PLAIN SIGHT

My personal experience examples of what this may look like.

Opening Story: Oxytocin Problem was Always There

Sometimes, we don't know what we are looking at. But once it is found, if we look backwards, it was clearly there the whole time. As I mentioned throughout this book, it was difficult because I didn't always know what I was looking for. We tend to try to look for the Bad Guy causing the problem, give it a name, and let it set up residency in our body. Because that was just the way it was. We attributed it to something or simply as a freak of nature. Looking back, I was amazed at how far back I could look and see the lack of one particular Good Guy being there all along: oxytocin. I also did not realize a Bad Guy could mimic it or impact my spleen the way it did.

Long story short, all six of my kids had to be caesarean delivery. The first two failed to progress at all, even with Pitocin (artificial oxytocin). The next four were just scheduled out. Here is the kicker, which had all medical staff and myself baffled, even with Pitocin, I could not feel my labor contractions or pain until I was in the high doses of Pitocin assistance. Hard to believe, I know. This should have been a clue, but I was just considered lucky.

The nurses would come walking by my labor room door and I would be playing cards with my husband. They would come look at the contraction monitoring machine. Yep, contractions three minutes apart. They would shake their heads and move onto the rooms with the screaming women who needed their help more.

Another scenario that was easier to brush off was how everyone has down days once in a while. What is considered more than normal? I never thought of it as depression because I did not feel depressed. I just felt tired... all the time.

Twenty plus years later, my pituitary gland problem was discovered. Oxytocin and the pituitary glands are a working team. It still did not register that the lack of this Good Guy was because a Bad Guy was occupying its seat. My body saw no need to make more. There was some there already, or so it thought.

Bear in mind, I don't think just taking oxytocin would have ever fixed my problems. Taking human growth hormone shots didn't. In fact, it made my problems worse. Oxytocin probably would have done the same thing. Strontium did as well.

I had to reprogram my body for it. I think the reprogramming of the misinformation while taking it made all the difference. Oxytocin was a particularly difficult nesting batch for me. It had two Mimickers and was a part of a homogeneous batch. Easy, no. Doable, yes!

Overview

Just as there are always two sides to a story, maybe there are two ways to look at the health problems we have. We have what we know, and we have what we might know if we look at it from a different angle. Instead of looking at the body as attacking itself, maybe the angle of the body protecting itself would point to different roads—different answers. Maybe our bodies have been trying to tell us all along, but we just didn't realize the clues we were being shown.

I think we need to assume the body wants to be well and something is stopping it. I think we need to think backwards about symptoms. Instead of trying to determine which came first, just acknowledge they are connected and figure out the connection. Like a crying baby, if we assume it was always hungry when it cried, it won't end well. If we assume the body is turning on itself, I think the same.

Inflammation, candida, low metabolism, and allergic reactions, for me, have been a sign of sorting problems. If I addressed the sorting problem, even if it was manually, it corrected these issues. I suspect these aren't the only clues to the body needing a DISH. I think there are other signs as well. Other hints in history and daily life. Hints we may see but never thought much about before. I will share a few of those situations in this chapter. I will also share a few more personal experiences on a much deeper level.

Let's get going.

Topic 1: Is This Evidence of DISH?

What are the implications if I am on the right trail here? Maybe I have missed the mark for the specifics of the why, but the *how* has shown results for me. I know the better I understood DISH, the more my health improved.

Fair enough, I understand why you would want more proof. I know just because it happened for me doesn't mean it's true for everyone. But maybe it is and we just don't see it because we weren't looking for it in this new way.

Have you ever seen those pictures that are really two pictures in one? Such as the psychological picture that shows an old woman and a young woman. One woman would be visibly obvious, while the other one may need to be pointed out before it is seen. It was always there, but we just didn't know what we were looking for to see it. Once we see it, it can't be unseen. Equally true is if you can't see it even when it's pointed out to you, you may never see it.

Our Surroundings Affecting Our Health

Are we seeing a manual DISH working here without realizing it?

***Modern Day*:** Back before the world had changed due to COVID-19, I had had experience with visiting my mom in the Intensive Care Unit (ICU) and my newborn son in the Neonatal Intensive Care Unit (NICU). For the ICU, the hospital she was at only allowed her to have one visitor at a time, but it could be a different visitor each time, just for a limited amount of time, usually fifteen to thirty minutes. Why? The nurse's words, decades ago, was it makes a difference and affects the patient *somehow*.

From my experience with NICU, only one person could see my son at a time and there could only be four visitors, period. The only exception was a pastor or other religious authority who would come in to pray for him. Was the denial of free entry to see him because of germs or was there more to it than that?

When we were talking to one of our son's doctors during this time, he commended us for coming every day. He said the babies that never make it are the ones the parents don't come in to visit. Yes, coming in doesn't guarantee he will make it, but it will guarantee he at least had a chance. Was it just emotional connections or were we giving off frequencies he needed?

A common practice in this NICU at the time was a method called Kangaroo Care. It appeared this was a BIG GOAL for the nurses. It helped the babies. Kangaroo Care is basically the act of placing the infant skin to skin on a parent, grandparent, or sibling. This intimate contact helped. I understand there would be psychological benefits to this. But what if these family members were also helping the newborns with their DISH?

In the Past: Smallpox was known as the traveling man's disease. According to the book *Pox: An American History* by Michael Willrich, this is what caused many towns to be leery of outsiders. This disease was greatly feared. When a family member would contract smallpox, people were encouraged to remove the family member from the home in an effort to protect other household members. If they were removed from the home, they were more likely to die than if they stayed where they were.[68] And if they survived the disease, they would have the presence of pox on their bodies for the rest of their life. Were these pox scars a new DISH for the body? [69]

While infected with this virus, when a person was relocated, were those changes in the environment too much at once for the body to deal with? The person had to focus on the smallpox virus and all those combinations of the new environment with it, as well as the old environment he left behind. I have no way of knowing those answers, but those questions are worth considering.

---

[68] Willrich, Michael, *Pox: An American History.* (New York: The Penguin Press, 2011), 31.

[69] Willrich, *Pox, 27.*

Topic 2: Is This Food Allergies?

Allergies Backwards

Instead of looking at allergies as allergies, I saw them as triggers, and eventually triggers to batches. If I knew the allergen, I avoided it until I was ready to target it. But sometimes, unfortunately for me, something safe to eat one day was not safe to eat the next day or thereafter... until I realized batches. Understanding batches changed everything.

Food allergies cause inflammation. Let's not assume it is the food's fault. What if the food contained something that enabled the body to fight something, but it either did not have

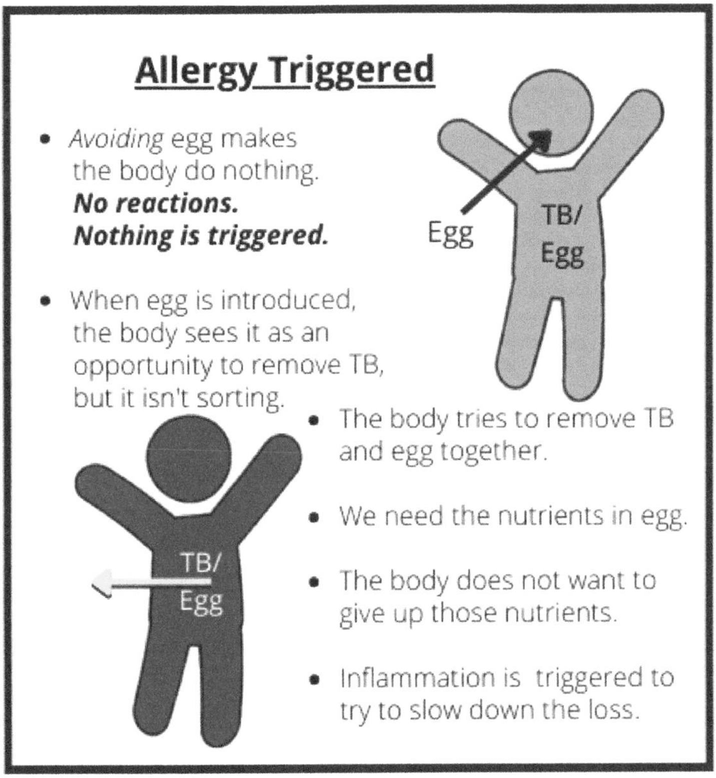
Allergy Triggered
• *Avoiding* egg makes the body do nothing. ***No reactions. Nothing is triggered.***
Egg
TB/ Egg
• When egg is introduced, the body sees it as an opportunity to remove TB, but it isn't sorting.
TB/ Egg
• The body tries to remove TB and egg together.
• We need the nutrients in egg.
• The body does not want to give up those nutrients.
• Inflammation is triggered to try to slow down the loss.

enough of the nutrient to finish the job or the nutrient(s) were attached to a Bad Guy? By being attached to this Bad Guy, eating what was needed to fight him caused the body to try to fight the combination. I understand, when having an allergic reaction to something, the body sends out Attacker cells to fight it. But something else—the need to keep the Good Guys in—may be going on as well.

Supplements Backwards

The reason we take supplements is because we need the nutrients in them. If the diet is bad, it may very well be just a Band-Aid. But if the diet is good, why is diet not enough?

- Why is diet AND supplements AND exercising not enough? There are many valid possibilities for this.
- What if we just entertain the thought that maybe something is awry with our body and its relationship with the nutrients running around in it?
- What if we are rejecting the nutrients through errant sorting?
- What if just holding these supplements is all we really need to do to get the levels to start going back up?

Our Diet

***Nutritional deficiencies*:** I know there is currently much talk about trace minerals being a key factor in managing our health. I also know if we are eating a Standard American Diet, it would be possible to not receive those nutrients. But if we are eating healthful and including those minerals in our diet, why are we not getting enough of them? A trace amount. That is so little. Why is nobody questioning this? Why are we not getting those minerals? Maybe we are, but our bodies are just disregarding these nutrients because it is failing to sort properly.

***Inflammatory foods*:** I know it is very, very difficult to think differently. I also know and did the avoiding of inflammatory foods to regain my health. I did it for over seven years. In the beginning, it did help. But I hit a wall that this diet would not let me climb over. I chose to not just stand and stare at the wall. There had to be a way over it.

With what I was learning about inflammation through experience, I rethought what I knew. I realized fragmented batches, wrong programming, and the nutrients present in these inflammatory foods were actually nutrients I needed in order to fight what my body was trying to fight. So, when I did consume them, my body saw this as an opportunity to fight. But the problem was that since the sorting was not happening correctly, the body also wanted me to not fight it as well. Tug-of-war, aka inflammation.

A Fixed DISH

The more misinformation I corrected, the stronger my DISH became, the less I needed to help it. The good food I ate was enough to do the job. An overall sense of well-being and the desire to get up and get moving and doing something, anything, had returned. I would have energy to spare. Body aches were gone. Basically, anything I was feeling because of nutritional deficiency was gone. I was no longer wasting my

Good Guys. This was the case regardless of the fact that I needed to manually do the DISH's jobs.

With a working DISH, the supplements and nutrients I took would help with the problem instead of contributing to it. The Good Guys were not at risk of being grouped with a Bad Guy (inflammation or nutrient depletion). If I needed medication for any reason, the medication would not only do its job, but maybe even reduce the risk of an inflammatory reaction. Trace amounts of the medication that seeped through into Lymph Land would be able to make their way to the surface of the skin and not become tied to the reason the medicine needed to be taken in the first place.

With the idea of symptoms stemming from deficiencies, I got to thinking. By having a working DISH, the body is able to sort its environment. Maybe this is why a person could be asymptomatic. Maybe the symptoms are brought on by the lack of needed Good Guys in the body. If the body is able to sort, it is not losing or becoming deficient in those Good Guys. Different deficiencies affect different areas of the body. Is it safe to say, if the deficiency isn't there, the symptoms are not either? If the Good Guys aren't getting grouped with the Bad Guys, the inflammation isn't there. The body is fighting what it is fighting without being affected, without showing symptoms. Just a thought.

Topic 3: Is This Multiple Sclerosis?

Something to think about...

I would like you to join me now in a quick Google search. (These are all screen shots.) I want you to see what I unearthed about multiple sclerosis in light of a faulty DISH. Let's take a look at what we already know and put it through this filter of needing a DISH.

A. More common in women:[70]

> It's a fact that more women than men are diagnosed with MS, but the reason why has left scientists scratching their heads. According to the National Multiple Sclerosis Society, "MS is at least two to three times more common in women than in men, suggesting that hormones may also play a significant role in determining susceptibility to MS.
>
> www.healthline.com/health-news/why-do-more-women-than-men-get-ms-051414
>
> Study Explains Why MS Is More Common in Women than in Men

B. Environmental trigger:[71]

> In addition to rheumatoid arthritis, the Epstein-Barr virus is closely linked to multiple sclerosis, inflammatory bowel disease, type 1 diabetes, juvenile idiopathic arthritis, and celiac disease.

---

[70] Burtchell, Jeri. "Study Explains Why MS Is More Common in Women Than in Men." Healthline. 20 October 2018. https://www.healthline.com/health-news/why-do-more-women-than-men-get-ms-051414.

[71] Shomon, Mary. "Causes and Risk Factors of Autoimmune Disease." Verywell Health. Updated 9 November 2021. https://www.verywellhealth.com/autoimmune-diseases-causes-risk-factors-3232655.

C. About the Epstein-Barr virus (EBV):

- EBV is a part of the herpes family and it is one of the top ten STDs.
- Childhood trauma, especially sexual abuse, has been linked to multiple sclerosis as well.
- I think one could reasonably guess that maybe an STD (STI) was acquired during this unfortunate time.

The top 10 STDs that are mostly seen are as follows:

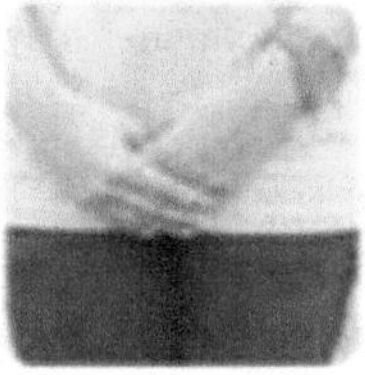

- Genital shingles (Herpes Simplex)
- Human papillomavirus (Genital warts)
- Hepatitis B.
- Chlamydia.
- Chancroid (Syphilis)
- Clap (Gonorrhea)
- Human immunodeficiency virus/Acquired immunodeficiency syndrome (HIV/AIDS)
- Trichomoniasis (Trich)

More items...

M https://www.medicinenet.com › article

What Are the Top 10 STDs? 4 Curable STDs, Spread & Safe Sex

The Mayo Clinic website states that "Many STIs have no signs or symptoms (asymptomatic). Even with no symptoms, however, you can pass the infection to your sex partners."[72]

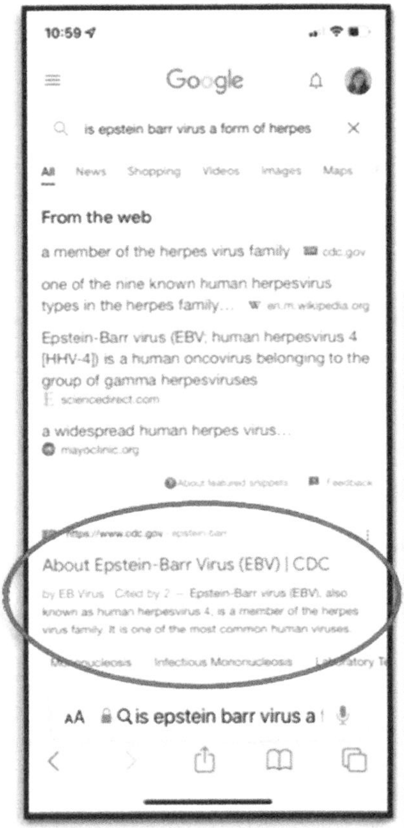

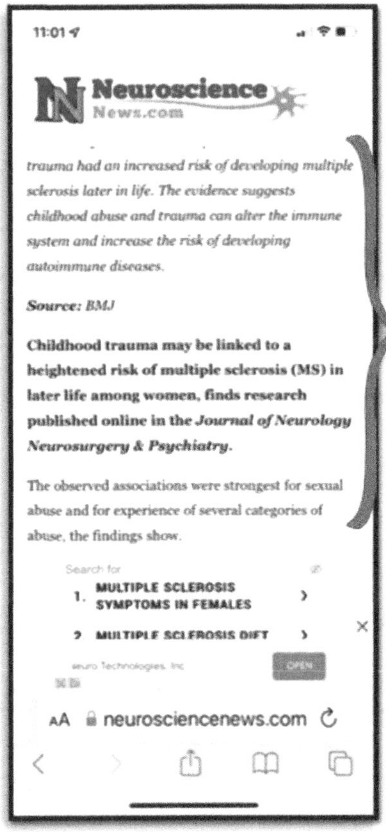

[72] Mayo Clinic Staff. "Sexually Transmitted Disease (STD) Symptoms." Mayo Clinic. 5 May 2022. https://www.mayoclinic.org/diseases-conditions/sexually-transmitted-diseases-stds/in-depth/std-symptoms/art-20047081.

D. Oxytocin Factor:[73]

Can this be translated as women NEED more oxytocin than men or lose more oxytocin than men? If they produce more, it's probably because they need more.

Do Men and Women Experience Oxytocin Differently?

Women typically have higher oxytocin levels than men.[7] (It's a key hormone involved in childbirth and lactation, after all). Biological differences aside, men and women appear to experience oxytocin in many of the same ways. It facilitates bonding with children, increases romantic attachment, and plays an important role in reproduction for both sexes.

E. Pantothenic Acid:[74]

Something caused my body to stop communicating properly. Was it because I was rejecting B5? Looks like that to me.

4. Maintains Healthy Nerve Function

Vitamin B5 is responsible for helping with nerve function, specifically for creating an important molecule called acetylcholine. The nervous system depends upon acetylcholine. This is the primary chemical that allows your nervous system to communicate back and forth with your organs.

Acetylcholine makes it possible for your brain and spinal cord to send nerve signals to our immune system, heart, lungs, kidneys, spleen, liver and more. It is also used to send nerve signals to muscles, so without enough pantothenic acid, nerve damage and impairment in movement can develop.

This is why one of the primary signs of a serious B vitamin deficiency is muscle impairment and pain, including a condition known as burning feet syndrome. This occurs when a person experiences lack of feeling in the feet along with painful burning, inflammation, and the feeling of ongoing fatigue and weakness.

---

73 Owens, Alexandra. "Tell Me All I Need to Know About Oxytocin." Psycom. 23 September 2021. https://www.psycom.net/oxytocin.

74 Levy, Jillian, CHHC. "Vitamin B5/Pantothenic Acid Deficiency & How to Get Enough!" Dr. Axe. 11 September 2021. https://draxe.com/nutrition/vitamin-b5/.

F. DISH:

Was the body failing to sort?

- Did something cause the frequencies of B5, oxytocin, and this virus to combine to where they could not separate from each other?
- Did this system failure cause the hormone women need more than men to deplete to where I could not fight the virus anymore without depleting it too low?
- Did this reduction in B5 cause the missing information to happen?
- Does this happen to more people than just me?

G. What I Determined:

I finally narrowed my problem down. Whenever I tried to fight my virus, my oxytocin and B5 levels would drop and not recover after supplementing them. This told me I had encountered a homogeneous batch: oxytocin, a virus, and B5.

The difficult part here was oxytocin was also being mimicked by a different Bad Guy.

H. What I Did:

I focused my efforts on the outside and inside of my body in small steps.

THE OUTSIDE:

- I had been taking B5, so I had some with me already.
- I bought an oxytocin spray.
- I carried both around in my pocket continually.

➢ Occasionally I would use a diluted form of the spray on my face, on the back of my neck, or both.

➢ I would also occasionally sprinkle some of the B5 capsule contents on the top of my head. It only required a trace amount. Not visible.

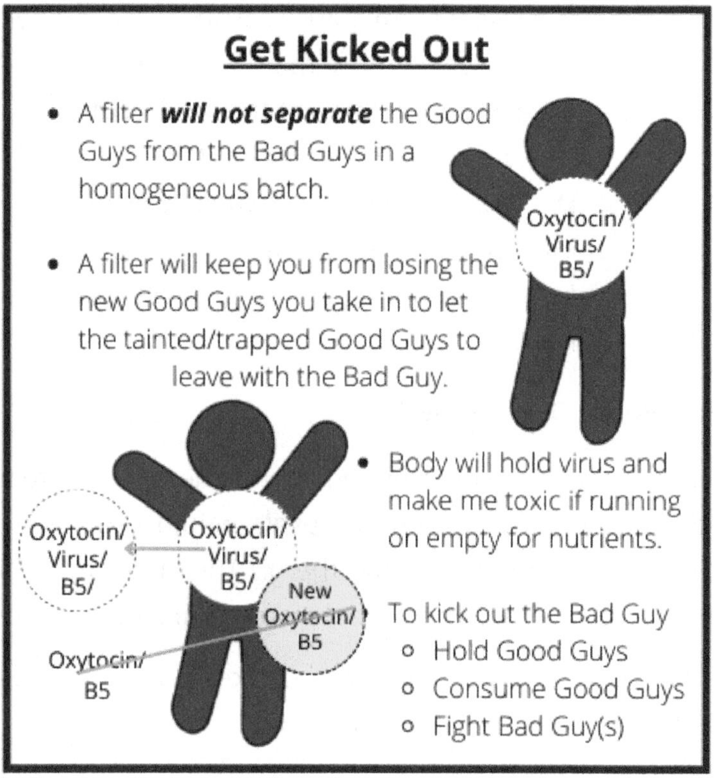

Get Kicked Out
A filter *will not separate* the Good Guys from the Bad Guys in a homogeneous batch.
A filter will keep you from losing the new Good Guys you take in to let the tainted/trapped Good Guys to leave with the Bad Guy.
Oxytocin/ Virus/ B5/
Body will hold virus and make me toxic if running on empty for nutrients.
Oxytocin/ Virus/ B5/
Oxytocin/ Virus/ B5/
New Oxytocin/ B5
Oxytocin/ B5
To kick out the Bad Guy
Hold Good Guys
Consume Good Guys
Fight Bad Guy(s)

THE INSIDE:

➢ **Before I ate…**

- If I was not eating anything with B5, I would take some of the supplement B5. (Frequency mattered more than quantity because it was a homogeneous batch.)
- I would take a prescribed supplement for oxytocin as well.

- I would also take either elderberry liquid or a turmeric supplement to help fight the virus I was activating by giving my body enough nutrients to cause it to try to kick the virus out.

➢ **After I ate…**

- At some point during the day, I would need to hold virus detox supplement for twenty minutes to three hours (to keep lymph roads open); it varied.
- Eventually, this would need to be done on each meridian clock segment.

➢ **Daily…**

- When fighting this virus, it appeared to have a very base Byproduct, or its leaving was exposing something very base. I occasionally needed to take an acid supplement for this. (See Appendix B for pH level information.)
- Be mindful when killing off a virus, the blood cell is killed with it. I needed to be taking the supplements required to help me to rebuild blood, including drinking plenty of mineral-rich water.
- I also made sure whatever supplements I was taking I was holding as long as necessary (3Ps Mode on page 196).
- I also wanted to keep the lymph roads open.
  - ✓ Soaking in tub with Epsom salt and a few drops of cinnamon essential oil.
  - ✓ Keep the lymph moving (walk or bike daily).

And, of course, the simple but not easy concept of everything connected. This was just one *top* point on *one of the main triangles*. So, there were other batches (triangles) that periodically needed to be dealt with throughout that were combined with this one. But always circling back to this one only.

For me, oxytocin was the Kingpin for this and two other major triangles. Between chlorobutanol being a Mimicker and this batch being homogeneous, there is no way I could have gotten past this without knowing what I know now about batches.

>> Sidenote About Elderberry Liquid <<<

Before taking this medicine

Ask a doctor, pharmacist, or other healthcare provider if it is safe for you to use this product if you have an autoimmune disease such as:

- multiple sclerosis;
- lupus; or
- rheumatoid arthritis.

Does this matter because a virus is tied to essential nutrients in the body?[75] *Evidently, somebody knows vitamin B is needed.*[76]

Still, many doctors say it's safe to take elderberry as part of a healthy **diet plan** that includes foods with vitamin B, **vitamin B6**, and **vitamin E**.

---

[75] Multum, Cerner. "Elderberry." Drugs.com. 21 February 2023. https://www.drugs.com/mtm/elderberry.html#:~:text=If%20desired%2C%20you%20may%20mix%20elderberry%20liquid%20with,as%20directed%20away%20from%20moisture%2C%20heat%2C%20and%20light.

[76] Reviewed by Pathak, Neha, MD. "Elderberry." Nourish by WebMD. 21 September 2020. https://www.webmd.com/diet/elderberry-health-benefits.

>>> *Maybe* more specifically B5 & oxytocin? <<<[77]

www.verywellhealth.com › elderberry-for-colds-and

Elderberry: Benefits, Side Effects, Dosage, and Interactions

Health Benefits | Possible Side Effects | Dosage and Preparation | W

Many of elderberry's health benefits are linked to anthocyanins. These substances are said to: 1. Work by clearing the body of free radicals that damage cells at the DNA level1 2. Have antiviral properties that may prevent or reduce the severity of certain common infections 3. Have anti-inflammatory benefits, modulating the body's immune response2

See full list on verywellhealth.com

Occupation: Nutritionist, Journalist

Personal Examples

Pretty much this whole chapter was about personal examples, so I see no need to include more here. What I would like to include instead is a different type of example. When a baby is screaming or fussing, it is trying to communicate. We don't know what it wants. We try to figure it out. Sometimes we get lucky and get it right. When we do, we store that information in hopes of finding patterns so when we hear that particular cry again, we can test to see if it was for the same reason. If it is, chalk it up as a win.

I think this is what our bodies are doing too. Our body's job is to function properly. It wants to do that. It is trying to tell us something is wrong. It is crying and fussing and

[77] Lefton, Jennifer, MS, RD/N, CNSC, FAND. "What Is Elderberry? Touted for Several Uses, Including Treating and Preventing the Cold and Flu." Verywell Health. Last reviewed 27 March 2023. https://www.verywellhealth.com/elderberry-for-colds-and-flu-can-it-help-89559.

refusing to be consoled. We need to learn to listen. Maybe listen differently than we ever had before.

Maybe you are thinking it is impossible. Or maybe you are just questioning whether or not it is possible. Well, someone gave me a book once about infant potty training. I thought they were full of it. But I read the book. I wondered about what I read. I started looking for the signs the book talked about. They were there! Signs I had seen all the time before but never thought anything of them. I gave it a casual try and, low and behold, this particular type of fussing was because she did not want to go to the bathroom in her diaper. I wouldn't believe it if I hadn't seen it for myself.

Maybe inflammation, nutritional deficiencies, pain, fatigue, and the like are our bodies trying to communicate with us. Maybe we need to consider another possibility for this. A possibility that was never on our radar before. A broken DISH.

Listen, Look, Test, Act.

Action Steps Summary

Are our bodies telling us they want to be well? Are we not listening? We are experiencing allergies, inflammation, pain, and the like. Why?

- Listen to our bodies.
    - Damage/pain occurred when misinformation was happening.

  - Stopping the misinformation stopped the pain and fatigue.
  - The manual DISH was needed.
  - Taking and holding supplements strategically depending on the batch type made the needed frequency.
- Look for patterns to test.
  - Holding proximate Good Guys goes far.
  - Sometimes it is even enough because it is preventing errant programming from happening.
  - Keeping Good Guys in—by preventing them from being diverted to the lymphatic system—SOMETIMES is enough without needing to take them.
- Simplify the equation to locate the real problem.
  - Inflammation may not be the problem; it may just be the warning light to look for misinformation.
  - Nutritional deficiencies may be telling us we need to reprogram misinformation before missing information occurs.

Conclusion for Chapter 11

I know throughout this book I have been throwing many new ideas at you. I hope I have at least caused you to think about what we have always believed to be true—and may be true—although not the root. I know the closer I would get to the really Bad Guys, when my body was circulating the misinformation still, it would cause my body to power down. The weight would come on. My body would do anything it could to get me to not fight, to not lose too many Good Guys. But once the coating of the Good Guy(s) was available on the outside consistently, my body would reprogram the mixed information. It has fixed every time, so far.

I know there is an abyss of stuff I do not know. I know finding the Bad Guy is a lot of work. Sometimes it took me a very long time to finally figure out how the Good Guy and Bad Guy were confused. But it worked. So, even though it is hard work, I chose to do it because of the results.

I could not ever say definitively this particular Bad Guy was ________. It didn't really matter. What mattered most was freeing the Good Guy being held prisoner by it. With that being said, I just wanted to reiterate:

- The concepts I've shared in this book worked repeatedly over the years in many different scenarios.
- The hard part was finding the connections.
- The amazing part was that it worked every time once I figured out the connection and the type of batch I was dealing with.

Yes, it is a pain to have to manually sort all the time. It is no more work than having to eat a decent meal every day or exercise. It is what it is—a needed paradigm shift. So, are you interested in learning how to think backwards?

Will it work for everyone? I don't know.

It is, after all, a hypothesis.

DISH: Defensive Individual Shield Hypothesis

DISH has two jobs.

1. Shield the Body
2. Sort what the Body Encounters

When DISH is doing its job,
I am winning against my health challenges.
When it is NOT doing its job, I am losing.

♦ ♦ ♦ It's that simple. ♦ ♦ ♦

AFTER: Altering Fields to Enable Recovery

How I help DISH to do its jobs.

1. Correct Misinformation
2. Fill in Missing Information

I am manually able to do the jobs
for DISH until my body is able to
do it on its own again.

♦ ♦ ♦ *Doable, but not easy.* ♦ ♦ ♦

CHAPTER 12:
HOW TO THINK BACKWARDS

Different questions lead to different starting points, which lead to different results.

Opening Story: My Soap

Because this frequency of DISH is supposed to be always changing, and it wasn't doing it on its own, I sway tested everything. I was just trying to survive. There was so much I wanted to do; I needed my body to be on my team. Because of years of this, I don't even really think or ask my body anymore what it wants. It is more of a gut feeling sometimes. Recently, my process of narrowing down the culprit would not give me any answers. Bacterial? No. Viral? No. Radiation? No. And so on. All I could think of was a picture of blackness. Yes. What on earth did that mean? No clue. It kept showing up regularly as the problem. I don't even remember how or why I realized this blackness was carbon. It was a huge sway forward for yes when I did. Carbon is in many things!

Shortly after this revelation, I was about to clean myself up to get out of the tub. I felt the need to wash with my son's body wash instead of the one I usually used. Strange. I read the ingredients and it had methylene blue in it among other ingredients. However, the methylene blue ingredient stuck out in my mind because the color of blue has always been a large player in my health. I also saw a health book pop up on my phone about this methylene blue. I wonder. I typed just the words *carbon* and *methylene blue* into my phone. Up pops an article about how carbon is used to clean up methylene blue. Dang! Eureka. There it was. Let's put it backwards. I bet methylene blue will help with carbon.[78]

Holding and soaking in methylene blue has helped me incredibly with this blackness issue. Interestingly, I have not taken it orally yet. If taking it orally is only to get it to the surface of my skin, then holding it or soaking in it would do the same. Why introduce something into the system if I don't have to? Why add in more for the body to sort if it isn't sorting correctly yet? Baby steps.

Will I need to eventually take it orally? Maybe yes, maybe no. I'll wait and see if the sway test changes. So far, no. I trust it. It has earned my trust because of how long it was all I could rely on.

Overview

Make Healthy Living Work

By continually striving to manually keep my DISH up, I noticed the techniques and approaches in the past that didn't work would now work. For example, I had failed at seeing any

---

[78] Bokil, Shantini A., and Niraj S. Topare. "Removal of Methylene Blue Suing Activated Carbon Prepared from Waste Fruit (Orange) Peels." SpringerLink. 25 February 2022. https://link.springer.com/chapter/10.1007/978-981-16-6875-3_15.

results the first three times I tried to do the Master Cleanse.[79] The fourth time I tried, I periodically held many different supplements throughout the day on different places on my body. I went the whole ten days and afterwards, I was finally able to be in a car again, as a passenger and driver.

Many of my environmental sensitivities went away because of this cleanse. In the past, before DISH, doing the cleanse would trigger such a candida flare-up I was advised to stop. I now believe this flare-up was an effort to prevent me from rejecting the Good Guys when I was trying to reject the Bad Guys they were tied to.

Make Treatments Less Harmful

The first time I did a foot detox bath, I returned home and went to bed, unable to rise again the following day. Needless to say, it had made me very weak. It made my minerals too low in spite of taking the supplements afterwards to replenish those Good Guys. The second time I went to have a foot detox bath, I came armed. I held one Bad Guy and five Good Guys. I also asked to hold the packet of the supplements I was to take afterwards. During the soak, it seemed more effective. I could feel a sensation going up both of my inner legs. I also was only tired for a couple of hours and never needed to lie down.

What I do not know, nor have I experienced, is what would happen for chelation therapy or chemotherapy. Would holding onto supplements prevent the loss and damage done during these procedures so they can be less

---

[79] Glickman, Peter. *Lose Weight, Have More Energy and Be Happier in 10 Days: Take Charge of Your Health with the Master Cleanse.* (Clearwater, FL: PeterGlickman, 2005)

harmful? Or what if they took home the empty IV bag to touch periodically? Would doing this prevent the body from having to fight the Stranger (needed medicine) and the Bad Guy at the same time? I don't know. I am only writing about what I experienced. But it would be nice to know.

Topic 1: Going Against the Grain

Going Against the Grain

Because of what I figured out, I had to take a leap of faith. I had to realize what helped me could hurt me. If I rushed getting the Bad Guy out when the roads were already blocked, I would only make the situation worse. I would cause more *cars* to show up in an already existing *traffic jam*. What I mean here is the very item I was taking to get well will—if my body wasn't sorting—become combined with the Bad Guy. To prevent this from happening so I could fight the Bad Guy, I would keep the Good Guy in my energy field. I would give the Good Guy an *exit ramp*.

If I failed to do this, I would need to slow down the traffic. If I didn't, I would hurt myself. If I tried forcing the Bad Guy out and it was attached to a Good Guy, it would only make me more toxic and have more inflammation and swelling. My body would have an internal tug-of-war contest going on below the surface.

When talking with my medical partners, they would tell me I am too toxic. Agreed. But how to remove the Bad Guys, or whether or not to even do so in the traditional way, was a different story. It depended on what type of batch the Bad Guy was hanging out in.

Toxicity, inflammation, candida overgrowth, and low metabolism were all signs to me of a batch still wrongly programmed in my body. The normal ways would not work to fix me. I had already tried. It was difficult to explain to my practitioner; though we agreed on the problem, I could not consent to the answer. I knew if I went down the same road again, I would get the same results. A dead end. I needed to convince them and show them to please look down this other path with me. I had information on me and this new concept had to be included before deciding what to do.

Toxicity/Detoxing

If I had a batch containing a Good Guy(s) with the Bad Guy, detoxing to remove the Bad Guy would pull the Good Guy with it. This pulling would cause resistance in the body. It would retaliate with either candida, inflammation, swelling, or what I often called powering down. The body would slow down the metabolism to keep it from rejecting too much of the good nutrient.

Instead of focusing on detoxing, cleansing, or increasing my metabolism, I needed to find who the Good Guy was and just hold it. This would normalize the situation. My body would power up again. I would no longer need to detox using what is called *cleansers* or *pushers*. I would only need to use *binders* for what was being activated. This would buy me time to narrow down what type of batch I was dealing with.

For example, when my doctor placed me on prescription HGH (human growth hormone) shots for my pituitary gland, it stopped my free fall of my body deteriorating before my eyes. But it also brought on all the allergies, environmental sensitivity, and utter fatigue. But even while taking the HGH shots four times a week, in less than six months, I went from doing intense *Tae Kwon Do* workouts to barely being able to swim across the gym's tiny pool. Hindsight: I think this is because the Bad Guy was pulling so many Good Guys out with him. These injections were revving up my body to do this rejecting even faster.

With that prior knowledge and the concept of DISH, it came in handy on a different appointment. When I went to find what nutrient I needed, my nutritionist saw my thyroid was underactive. He wanted to give me something to boost my thyroid. I politely but emphatically declined. I had been going to him for years, so he was willing to listen to what I had to say. I convinced him to go at it from a different angle. He did. (BTW: Thank you so much, A.C.) It worked. It immediately fixed all the other problems showing up at the time.

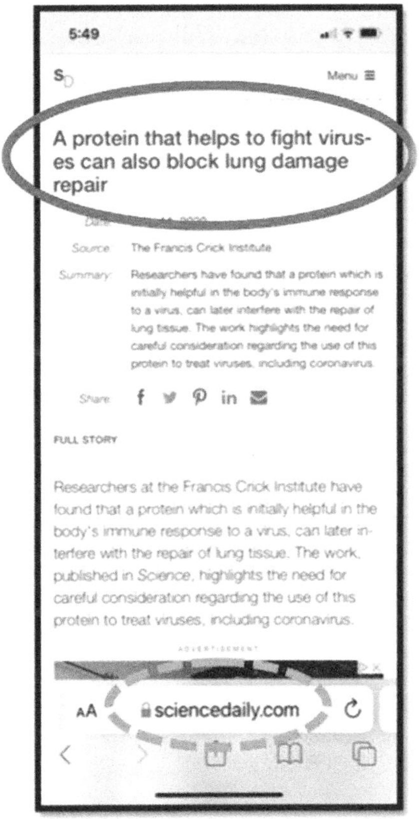

There are several examples I can give here, but what it narrows down to is if there is a batch that has not been separated out yet and it has good and bad together in it, forcing the bad out only hurt me more. The symptom of chronic inflammation was the desperate attempt for my body to slam on the brakes.

There Is Always Fallout

I alluded to this earlier about where it goes wrong. This could be in the form of supplements or food. If my DISH is not working, be it manually or automatically, what I am taking to fix my problem will ALWAYS become a part of the problem. I believe this is what is going on in this example I found online. It is a screen shot taken from my iPhone on April 18, 2022.[80]

What I am trying to tell you in this book I think can be seen in many places. Will you consider looking at the information you are given from a different angle? In the screen shot I just showed you, if the patients were holding the protein on a continuous basis, would that change everything? I truly believe so.

Getting Better

Sometimes there are necessary evils. If I were to have surgery, I definitely would want to be sedated and avoid bacteria growth. But it is even more than that. It could just be the foods or the nutritional supplements I was taking during this time. If the body isn't sorting, anything is game. Anything can become stuck together. This is why prevention is so key. Whatever I took to help me could become part of the problem if I did not keep it in my energy field for a period of time first. So simple. Why wouldn't I? Especially if it could make such a big difference.

---

[80] Francis Crick Institute. "A Protein That Helps to Fight Viruses Can Also Block Lung Damage Repair." ScienceDaily. 11 June 2020. https://www.sciencedaily.com/releases/2020/06/200611152453.htm.

But that is not all. The body makes hormones and chemicals when it is confronted with a Bad Guy. These can become attached and depleted as well. Cortisol. It is always associated with stress. But the body also makes cortisol when being attacked by a Bad Guy.[81] We need cortisol. Cortisol is our friend. (Sorry, kid's movie reference. I couldn't resist.) But if we have too much cortisol, it is a problem; if we don't have enough cortisol, it is a problem. This is an example of the body having symptoms of too much and not enough at the same time.

In my case, I opened up a capsule of Super Cortisol Support and sprinkled in a trace amount of the powder into a large glass spray bottle. I filled it with filtered water, shook it, and proceeded to spray it on my kidney(s). If I felt my anxiety building up in my body for no known reason, I assumed my body was making it to fight a Bad Guy. By spraying it on me, it was a win-win scenario. If I had excess cortisol tied to a Bad Guy, spraying it on gave me an exit for the cortisol to leave. If I was making excess cortisol to fight a Bad Guy, it prevented the cortisol from becoming attached to the Bad Guy it was fighting. Either way, the body would be able to correct its cortisol levels so I could continue to fight the problem.

Even as I write this, it sounds so crazy. How can it be that simple? But it is. Remember, this is something a person with a healthy DISH does without even being aware of it. I was just manually doing what my body couldn't so I could get back into the game of life. I guess it makes more sense than I thought.

---

[81] Author unknown. "Chapter 12.3 Stress & Health." Quizlet.com. Last accessed 27 March 2023. https://quizlet.com/15310181/chapter-123-stress-health-flash-cards/.

Topic 2: Ask Different Questions

Below are a few of the characteristics that I noticed went away once I fixed my DISH, so I am going to suggest (not assume) they were present because of my DISH being broken.

Candida and Inflammation: Is this a check engine light for my body?

Many of the symptoms associated with these are quite similar, so I'm going to group them together here. My body for some reason had turned on itself, or so it seemed. I think this was the body's attempt to power down. It needed to slow down the loss of nutrients or hormones. Candida sufferers usually have vitamin deficiencies: magnesium, essential fatty acids, vitamin B6, and a variety of other nutrients. The number one vitamin currently associated with inflammation reduction is vitamin D. I tried taking large doses of all these supplements. The symptoms never really went away. Was my body doing something to reject these nutrients?

When I held the proper supplements, my inflammation disappeared within hours. I was *making the equal sign* my body was failing to make. But in order for this to happen, it needed to be all the correct supplements, at the correct time, in the correct spot. Ugh, right?! Take heart, it's a learned skill.

Conflicting Test Results: Is the enemy's game plan being concealed?

I went to the doctor. He ran some tests for what he thought might be the problem based on his observations and analysis of my answers. The test results came back, and they were within the range of normal. Maybe a low normal, but normal.

Maybe not my normal, but normal. Well, that doesn't help much, does it?

Another incident that comes to mind is a documentary I watched about Lyme disease. Doctors were being threatened with losing their medical licenses because even if a test result for Lyme came back negative, this doctor was choosing to treat his patients for Lyme anyway. It didn't matter that his treatments were helping his patients to improve. The poor doctor's hands were tied.[82]

Are we relying too heavily on antibody testing when it can't tell us everything? It can tell us what we fought. It can't tell us if we are still fighting it. It is probably also possible the test cannot tell us if the body is too weak to fight the problem. What if this Lyme disease is a Mimicker of something the body needs, possibly brain related? Perhaps the body has chosen to stay with the enemy rather than kill off our brain! Thank you, body.

It is more about keeping the Good Guys in than getting the Bad Guys out.

Nutritional Deficiency: Are these deficiencies from my body rejecting them?

I can't count how many times I took large doses of what I was deficient in and the needle in the tank wouldn't even budge.

[82] Gravitas FREE MOVIES. *Under Our Skin (1:44:18). 25 July 2012. Online Video Clip. YouTube.* https://www.youtube.com/watch?v=2JgR_Jfbhv8.

(And yes, this was while on a gluten-free diet for those of you thinking this may have been the cause.)

Or I would have symptoms for too much AND not enough of the same nutrient. It was building up in my body, but my body could not utilize it.

Maybe malabsorption isn't the only problem. Maybe we are flat out rejecting them as well.

Health Issues with Organs: Which came first, the problem or the deficiency?

"Your (insert organ here) isn't working properly. You need more (insert Good Guys here)." What if the deficiency was because of the problem instead? What if the problem showed up, the body tried fighting it, there was too much inflammation, the Traffic Jam happened, thus the Vicious Cycle was started?

Sensitivity to Electricity or EMF: Is this a signal my body's shield is down?

I'm not sure how far along this would need to be in order to be considered bad before it is a factor. I know many claim to have challenges with this. Many products can be bought to protect yourself from EMFs. Some people may have never even heard of this problem before. If you have never experienced feeling physically ill after being exposed to electricity or radiation, you are probably like the fish in bowl A. You cannot relate to or possibly understand how on earth it's possible for this to be the problem. Well, we fish in bowl B see it differently.

The EMF may not be the illness, but it may be giving off enough energy to where I was the weaker one. By losing the *Energy Field War Game*, my body was having Bad Guys coming into my shield faster than I could remove them. I was unable to deflect anything. This inability to deflect and sort caused other physical symptoms to appear.

Strong Energy but Blocked Channels (Acupuncture): Is my body protecting itself?

My acupuncturist was frequently frustrated with this because she could tell my energy level was high but something, always something, rarely the same something, would be interfering with my meridians being open and flowing with energy.

Would the flowing of this energy cause misinformation to flow more frequently and hurt me more than the blocked channels?

New Food Allergies: Did I start the battle and retreat from lack of Good Guys?

I was never a fan of the Standard American Diet. The less packaging the better was a pretty safe motto to follow. I did have to go down the rabbit trail of a gluten-free, egg-free, dairy-free, soy-free, corn-free, artificial preservative-free diet. I was one hundred percent gluten free for five years; one hundred percent dairy and egg free for three years. But regardless of how many foods I avoided, the healthier I became, the more food allergies I would have. I know sunflower seeds are a pretty rare allergen food. Yep, allergic to them too. So, if you have ever been on a raw diet, try being on one when you are allergic to bananas, tomatoes, avocadoes, and sunflower seeds! Not cool.

Another possibility of an example of a broken DISH would be for a new food allergy to begin after an illness. I would definitely suspect the illness as being tied to the food because a nutrient in the food was helping me to recover from the illness. I think this may be why I was acquiring new food allergies daily.

Healthy Living Wasn't Working: Is this a sign of a broken DISH?

I know "healthy living" is a very broad category that can be interpreted differently by many people. I would like to generalize it as a person who is consciously and daily seeking out ways to improve their health and acting upon the information of the Big Five mentioned earlier.

Do the Big Five work only for those who have a working DISH?

If we are doing these five things and seeing no results, are we being hindered by a broken DISH?

Are we rejecting our Good Guys?

Are we holding onto our Bad Guys?

Do we need to make a manual DISH so the Big Five will start working for us?

Clinically Depressed: Are we rejecting hormones because of misinformation?

This was frustrating to me. I was told I was clinically depressed. I did not feel any of the emotional symptoms I would group with depression. Yes, my body was tired, so tired. I was frustrated, so frustrated. I knew something wasn't working right and I felt like nobody was listening. Each practitioner had their box or their known cure for whatever ailed me. Did it work? Nope. Was this caused by a nutrient deficiency? It's known to happen.

One particular time sticks out vividly in my mind. At one of my follow-up visits to my doctor, I was talking with her about the symptoms I was having. Her words: "Well, that doesn't make any sense. It shouldn't be doing that." "It" being the diagnosis she had given me. So, instead of thinking that MAYBE it was a misdiagnosis, she made me feel like she thought I was lying about the symptoms I was having. I did not want more medicine. I did not want *any* medicine. How could I benefit from lying to her?

So, basically, I was being told I had an illness I had no symptoms for, but what I had symptoms for did not have an illness associated with it. So, when a person is called a liar, it is easy to get angry. What was their conclusion? "Ah, see, getting angry is a symptom for this ailment we think you have." Circular reasoning or idiot loop? Didn't really matter. I just knew I was stuck, and I didn't want to be. I also knew I wasn't going to find any answers with them. I was talking and nobody was listening.

Difficulty Removing Parasites: Are they protecting me from something?

Parasites. Disgusting. Gross. Not something I would want anybody to know I had. Embarrassing, too, but they shouldn't be. I didn't do anything out of the ordinary to be cursed with this problem, but cursed I was. They had taken up residency with a very strong foothold. Was the reason for this stronghold because of all the other problems I had? Not because the problems made me weaker but because the problems would have hurt me more.

Were my parasites and I in a mutually beneficial situation? Did the parasite feeding on the inflammation protect me from the inflammation? Or did I create too much inflammation fighting them in Lymph Land to where there was a traffic jam? Are they now tied to an essential Good Guy? Is my body in a tug-of-war scenario waiting for the correct information to update the circulating errant information?

Two-Year Marker: Was my body too weak to fight a Bad Guy in the past?

I know this sounds pretty vague, but as I said before, I'm not saying this is how it is. I'm just sharing observations I have seen. When talking with other individuals who have been diagnosed with panic attacks, I noticed a pattern I believe warrants further investigation. But alas, I do not have the resources to do this. About two years after surgery on an injury that required strong painkillers, the first panic attack shows up. Did wrong programming occur because of a broken DISH two years earlier? Did the need for the painkillers in the first place create a perfect storm for the Danger Zone to be present as I discussed in Chapter 5? I can't help but wonder if the kidneys or liver were unable to handle the load of the medication given. If that is the case, is it possible for a problem to slip through and the errant information to now circulate throughout the body? Circulating for two years causing a significant amount of the blood in our bodies to contain this mistake.

Noise Bothered Me: Am I trying to limit my exposure to other frequencies?

If I were to Google *noise bothers me*, it would talk about the person being on high alert as the reason for it. I could see that. However, frequencies are frequencies. Noise is a frequency. Is it possible this noise was affecting me more on a frequency health level? Was this extra frequency combined with the other frequencies I was already working on just a little too much for my body to handle? Because my sorting system was malfunctioning, was I unable to sort all those frequencies down into bite-size pieces? Was my DISH unable to do its first job of deflecting most of them?

Topic 3: Focus on Good Guy(s)

We have been taught to read labels. Read labels in search of Bad Guys. Well, now it is backwards. My body knows it is supposed to remove Bad Guys. In a perfect world, I wouldn't have to worry much about them. But we don't live in a perfect world. Ideally, I would just prevent the Bad Guys from coming in. Sometimes I can't control this. When I can't avoid it, I remember the Good Guys. I strive to prevent the Vicious Cycle. I read labels looking for Good Guys. This way if my DISH wasn't working, I could do it manually. I could provide an exit for the Good Guys, at least.

Protect the Good Guys: Prevention is far more effective than correcting.

- Avoid the problem in the first place.
    - Hold the Good Guys present in the ingredients of medication I am taking.
    - Hold proximate Good Guys of the targeted organ during times of inflammation.
    - Hold proximate Good Guys for detox organs if currently having challenges with my DISH.
- Focus on keeping the Good Guys around.
    - Food dislikes may reveal a needed nutrient being rejected when consumed.
    - A food craving may reveal there is missing or misinformation.
    - If craving something not necessarily good for me:
        - Read the ingredients list.
        - What is my body trying to tell me?

- ✓ For example, crave cola > my body needed phosphorus.

Find the Good Guys: How do I find what Good Guys were needed or being affected?

- ➢ Use the methods of how the batches are formed to narrow down possible Bad Guys, if possible.
  - o Hold the Good Guy if there is a known Bad Guy who mimics or wants to occupy the same spot of a Good Guy.
  - o Examples:
    - Strontium 90 vs. good strontium
    - Aluminum occupies calcium channels[83]
    - Chlorabutanol vs. oxytocin
- ➢ Learn what Good Guys different organs need.
  - o If I was taking in the Good Guys and still deficient, do I need to do a batch neutralizing session?
  - o Is there a Bad Guy or its Byproduct, copying a Good Guy?
    - If so, help the body to recognize the difference between the two, via missing information or misinformation.
      - ✓ For me, Byproduct of Lortab copied testosterone.
      - ✓ For me, Byproduct of pesticide mimicked progestogen.

---

[83] Health Matters. "Aluminum." Health Matters. Last accessed 27 March 2023. https://healthmatters.io/understand-blood-test-results/aluminum.

- Give the Good Guys an escape route.

➢ The opposite is true as well. If I had a particular organ causing problems, what Good Guys could I put in my manual DISH to help the organ keep the Good Guy levels up?

The problem wasn't found until I knew

which Good Guy(s) was being impaired and how.

Keep in mind the size of the batches (triangles). I couldn't run off and hold all of these items at once. The batch (triangle) would be too big. It would have caused too many Bad Guys to leave at once. I cannot tell them to leave until I am manually making the DISH of the Good Guys. The body needed time to become stronger and recover. Let the Good Guys build up reinforcements for a while before leveling up.

I know. It sucked to go slow, but I needed to let my body decide how fast I could go because I had decades of debris, I needed to finally flush out.

I have enclosed a partial chart as an example of what it may look like to try to find the Good Guys I needed. To fill in this chart, I mainly focused on how batches are formed. I also considered Good and Bad Guys as possibilities.

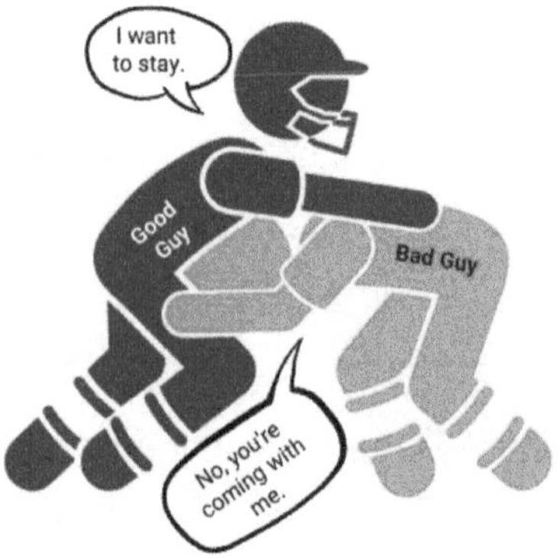

Know Contaminant: Strontium-90		Exposure	Proximity	Resemblance
	BAD GUY	Lead vest Potassium Iodine needed, drank for MRI Other Camp Lejeune contaminants*	Cerium—present naturally with radiation, catalyst to refine petroleum Vanadium—used in nuclear reactors	Cobalt-60—some medical X-ray machines Cobalt in jet fuel Potassium-40
	GOOD GUY	Potassium Iodine	Strontium (bones) Cerium—used for making collagen (everywhere body needs collagen [lungs, brain, intestines, etc.]) Iodine (thyroid) Vanadium (spleen)	Good Strontium Good Cobalt Good Potassium

*I even did a batch with dog and concrete. I had read bags of dog carcasses labeled radioactive were found at Camp Lejeune when a parking lot was going to be repaved. This information was actually very helpful. I no longer have an aversion to dogs.

Know Contaminant: Vinyl Chloride (polymer)		Exposure	Proximity	Resemblance
	BAD GUY	Other Camp Lejeune contaminants	PVC pipes for water supply	Chlorine > anything containing chlorine PVC pipes Polyester Acrylic
	GOOD GUY	Collagen	For making collagen: vitamin C, zinc, copper, sulfur Places in the body needing collagen	Chlorine Gelatin

Know Contaminant: Chlorinated hydrocarbons		Exposure	Proximity	Resemblance
	BAD GUY	Dry-cleaning solution Industrial solvent Pesticide Other Camp Lejeune contaminants	Pharmaceuticals	Chlorine > anything containing chlorine Carbon > anything containing carbon
	GOOD GUY	Lipids (cells, organs & tissues)	Body is affected everywhere	Methylene blue Chlorine Carbon: Basic building block to form proteins, carbohydrates, and fats.[84]

✓ Notice there is overlapping of items.

✓ The information looks overwhelming.

✓ But it really isn't if we remember how batches are formed.

✓ I'll explain more in the next diagram.

[84] Singer, Glenn. "What Does Carbon Do for Human Bodies?" azcentral: Part of the USA Today Network. Last accessed 27 March 2023. https://healthyliving.azcentral.com/carbon-human-bodies-4307.html.

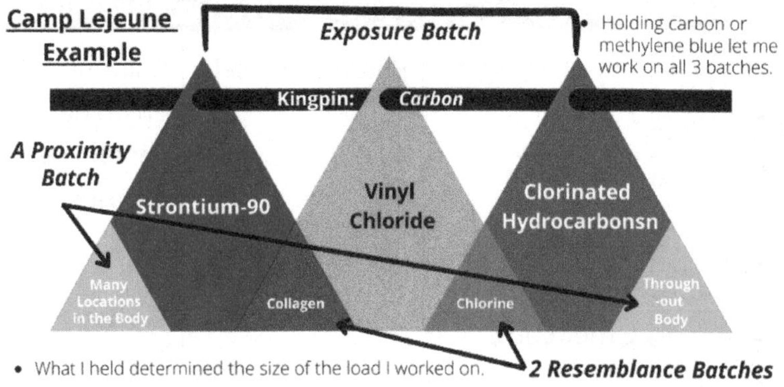

Use the Good Guys: *Only give the body what it can handle.*

- ➢ Controlling the DISH manually controls the size of the batch.
- ➢ Want body to have time to process out Bad Guys.
- ➢ Want body to have time to rebuild.
- ➢ Targeting one will trigger others as the body feels stronger.
  - o Holding methylene blue or carbon would make me work on all batches. Don't want to do this too soon.
  - o Better to hold collagen and chlorine alternately first.
  - o I was alternating between strontium and vinyl chloride when I started taking supplements high in chlorine.
    - Taking the supplements made me more toxic because it was forcing me to start fighting chlorinated hydrocarbons.
    - Making a manual DISH for chlorinated hydrocarbons allowed me to continue fighting the first two without becoming toxic or having inflammation.

Personal Examples

My kidneys had been hurting, again. It wasn't my kidneys though. It was the load my kidneys needed to process out. I had been given a dozen different supplements over the past few months to try to help my kidneys heal and do their job more efficiently. But they were still getting hurt. They weren't only hurting but getting worse. It appeared like my body was removing Bad Guys at an alarming rate. My engine (kidneys) was in overdrive without enough oil to keep the gears lubed. I needed to find the lubricant my kidneys needed instead of trying to continually fix the damaged gears.

I chose to learn about how the kidneys worked exactly. I watched a YouTube video that explained how they functioned.[85] It was fascinating. With this information, I chose my supplement of choice, Himalayan pink salt, from the supplements recommended to me in the past. I had been taking this supplement for some time. It helped, until it didn't. Since I had been holding it in my energy field when taking it, I suspected this was not enough. Plug the holes. I taped the supplement on the area by both kidneys.

> *Sidenote: Regardless of how the problem was caused (exposure, proximity, or resemblance), step one of holding or "plugging holes" with the item would fix it as long as it did not turn into a homogeneous or Mimicker batch.*

---

[85] Institute of Human Anatomy. "Why Drinking Water Is So Important." (00:15:33) 10 December 2021. Online Video Clip. YouTube. https://www.youtube.com/watch?v=-slnr4TGA4Y.

Doing this simple step drastically reduced the amount of healing supplements and pink salt I needed to be taking. Granted, I had to do this for almost six months. It is like my body trusted me to do the sorting so it was going full speed ahead. If I quit the sorting, my body was still pressing on. I would need to immediately get the salt back on me again.

If you are still wondering if it is an absorption thing, I thought you would like to know I taped it on the waistband of my clothing. The salt never came into direct contact with my skin.

Doing this simple step not only lubricated the hypothetical gears I was talking about, but it was like I also added the high-octane fuel as well. It caused my body to be more effective. I needed to hold metal detox and virus detox (Byproduct remedies) periodically for months even though I was not taking anything to specifically remove heavy metals or to fight the virus.

If I would start feeling worn down, I would wonder why and then remember the pants I had on did not have the pink salt on them. Fixing that, fixed it.

After the six months, I would just sprinkle a little on my head every day. It was enough.

How can it be that simple?

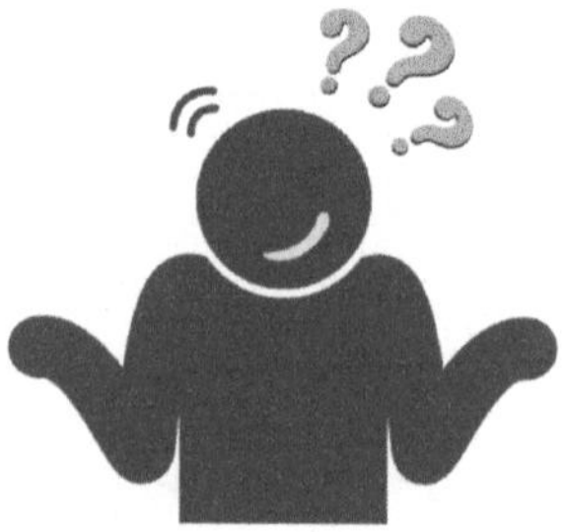

Action Steps Summary

What would it look like backwards?

Instead of focusing on who the Bad Guy was, I focused on finding and keeping the Good Guys in. Even though I was doing the healthy lifestyle, these Good Guys were seriously low in numbers.

- I assumed my body wanted to be well.
- When something went wrong, I would consider what my body may be trying to tell me.
- I focused on the Good Guy needed for my body to fight the battle itself.
- I assumed any inflammation or nutritional deficiencies were warning lights, not the problem.

Ask different questions

Think about the "what came first, the chicken or the egg" scenario. Yes, the problem is present. Suggesting it isn't the main problem is not the same as suggesting there isn't a problem.

- Is my body sending a warning light?
- Is my body trying to tell me I was failing to sort something?
- Is my body trying to create a DISH?
- Is it possible my body was missing information?
- How can I protect my organs so they are able to do their job properly?

Create a manual DISH

- I assumed the broken DISH was the problem.
  - Sway test to find how I needed to adjust my DISH frequency.
  - Investigate why this was the case.
    - ✓ Look for missing information.
    - ✓ Look for connections.
- Altering what was in my energy field altered the size of the batch I was doing.
- Only have my body work on the size of the batch it could handle.
  - Allow my body time to remove Bad Guys.
  - Allow my body time to rebuild.

Conclusion for Chapter 12

In order to be able to think backwards, it was almost like living in an opposite world. All this inflammation and the nutritional deficiencies causing so many health problems are definitely there. Realizing this, the tendency would be to search out and find the Bad Guy. Understandable. It has always been the case. But maybe we need to look at these issues like they are the warning signs, not the problem.

For me, sometimes I knew who the Bad Guy was. However, I only used this information to find what Good Guy was being harmed. Sometimes I needed to guess who the Bad Guy was. Guessing would get me close to finding the Good Guy needed. I may know it was a virus, but I may not know what type of virus it was. It didn't really matter. The Good Guy is the end goal. Keeping him in my body so my body could do what it was meant to do. Keeping the inflammation and nutritional deficiencies as a nonissue by manually doing my DISH's job.

- We study the Bad Guys to find what Good Guys are being harmed.
- We deal with the Bad Guys only when absolutely necessary based on what type of batch they are in.
- We focus on keeping the Good Guys in.
    - Watch for proximity challenges during inflammation.
    - Watch out for Mimickers.
- We assume the body knows what it is supposed to be doing, and if it is not, it is a warning light.
    - Misinformation—wrong sorting caused missing information.
    - Missing information—deficiency caused a glitch.

Conclusion

Key Takeaways for This New Perspective

CONCLUSION: THE DIFFERENT PERSPECTIVE

Helping our bodies to do what they were meant to do.

Opening Story: Finding a Helper

I am aware of health challenges associated with malabsorption. In fact, it was the reason I went to see a naturopath for the first time. I had gone gluten free. I lost thirty pounds in the first three months of doing so. I also read about how some damage may have occurred from this being undiagnosed over a long period of time. I figured I should check to see if this was the case for me since it made such a difference in my health. I thought maybe it was why I plateaued. I felt much better initially, but it, too, tapered off. The needle on my engine would never hold. I had a slow leak somewhere. But where? Not only did my energy taper off, but my body also started adding more allergies to my arsenal on a daily basis. My naturopath doctor put me on many supplements. Some at very high doses. Did it work? You guessed it. Nope.

I am also aware that when the body is deficient, it is deficient. We need to replenish. But are we trying to fill up a bucket with a hole in it? This is the case when the body is rejecting what it should be accepting. I believe this happens when the sorting system lever is flipped to "off." On many occasions, I was trying to fill up my bucket (body) while having holes (sorting system not working) in it.

When I really started understanding what this sorting system was doing, I was able to plug those holes. I realized this sorting malfunction was causing me to reject essential Good Guys in my body. Trying to explain this to my doctor without sounding crazy was difficult. For me, I went to the same nutritionist doctor for about a year trying to translate what he was telling me into my own process. I finally got up enough nerve one day after he muscle tested me. He said my body was low in HCL (betaine hydrochloride), a Good Guy I didn't even know existed. I just now knew he was a needed Good Guy regardless of his job.

I asked him a question. I said, "Is it low or is my body rejecting it?" It came back as rejecting. He shook his head and said he didn't even know what to think about it. He had never heard of it. My appointment time was up, but I left the office with hope for a change.

The following month, I focused on trying to figure out a way to share with him the most information I could in the shortest amount of time. I needed him to help me figure out what to do next. So many nutrients and hormones, so little time. If he could be open to my input, I would rather ask and get help than try to figure all these supplements out on my own. You see, he knew more about *the* body and what it needed to function. He knew many things I did not. But I knew what *my* body was doing, and everything he told me to do HAD to be filtered through that.

I knew he had a hard time wrapping his head around the idea of me usually holding the supplements instead of taking them. I was challenging his whole world of knowledge. But he saw it working.

Was I disregarding the Big Five? No. I was, however, looking at them differently. I was trying to get myself into the group of people who actually benefited from the Big Five.

Overview

Have you ever heard the saying "like cures like"? It is the mantra homeopathic participants are most known for. It is the belief that an illness can be corrected by exposing oneself to something that would cause the same symptoms of what they were experiencing. However, this is not unique to homeopathy. It actually originated with Hippocrates (460–377 BC), the Father of Medicine. Even modern medicine follows this same basic philosophy. If you were to get a vaccination, you are giving yourself the virus, part of the virus, or something similar to it. From what I can see, both of them have the same concept in mind, but implement it very differently. However, the common ground is "like cures like."

"By similar things a disease is produced and through the application of the like is cured." —Hippocrates

---

The DISH concept is an extension of this belief as well. Maybe it isn't just an extension though. Maybe it is the missing piece to why a treatment sometimes worked and sometimes didn't. Maybe we just needed to add one more piece in order for it to work better.

My doctor and my homeopath were both on the right path for my health. However, neither could help me get my life back. Figuring out DISH and applying what I learned about it, combined with what they told me, I was able to improve.

Improve enough to where my pituitary gland is now a nonissue.

When it comes to the sliding scale of medical philosophy, maybe any approach could or would work better if we just factor in the possibility of a broken DISH. Maybe the people who are falling through the cracks just need to manually do their DISH's jobs for a while. Maybe...

Topic 1: The Big Five Backwards

If the reason the Big Five is frequently ignored is because it doesn't work for everyone, maybe realizing there are two types of people will make a difference here. Maybe creating the DISH manually for the second group will enable them to be a part of the first group.

The Big Five Health Challenges Through the Eyes of DISH

1. **Why Diet:** Nutrition matters.
    - We can't get better if we don't have the Good Guys to do their job.
    - Quantity doesn't matter if there are leaks.
    - Those leaks could be from different possibilities.
        - Using up—they are doing their job.
        - Rejecting—trapped in a batch.
2. **Why Exercise:** A healthy body is a moving body.
    - Lymph moves in a moving body.
    - Lymph being bogged down is a recipe for disaster.
        - Lymph Land getting too crowded is the Danger Zone.
        - Misinformation led to missing information.
        - Missing information led to the body malfunctioning.
    - When I didn't want to exercise.
        - Was it because misinformation would circulate more quickly?
        - Was I lacking the needed nutrients from rejecting them?

3. **Why Stress:** Need lower cortisol levels.
    - Stress is not the only source of cortisol.
    - Cortisol is needed for bodily function.
    - Cortisol may become stuck to the Bad Guy.
        - **Problem:** Cortisol unable to leave properly.
        - **Solution:** Make sure cortisol has an exit route.
4. **Why Avoid Bad Guys:** Make workload lighter on the organs.
    - Some Bad Guys are Mimickers of Good Guys.
    - When detox organs have too much to do, this is when the traffic jam occurs in Lymph Land.
5. **Why Avoid Inflammation:** Don't want body to attack itself.
    - See inflammation as the warning light instead of the problem.
    - Find out what Good Guy is being attacked, which is causing the inflammation to occur.
    - Stop the attack.

By realizing my DISH was what was broken, I used AFTER so what did not work before would now work. It enabled me to take the needed supplements I otherwise couldn't take. I focused on an equal sign instead of the problem. Granted, I had to continually change the DISH frequency manually, and yes, it is a pain in the butt to do so. More work. But it has given me my life back.

If I was working on a complete batch, I was able to exercise, or go places, or be in front of my computer, or be inside of my house with the electricity on. Stuff easy to take for granted. Stuff I enjoyed doing. However, my desire for self-preservation prevented me for years from participating in these activities.

Is it possible for a group A person to really understand us group B people? The weird decisions we make. The strange things we do. These are not based on weirdness but on the desire to survive. We continually analyze every event on how it would make us feel afterwards and whether it is energy well spent or better reserved for a different time.

Manually altering my DISH has enabled me to start making yes decisions more often based on what I want to do and not what I am able to do. Will I always have to manually sort my DISH? I don't know. I am grateful I don't have to wait until it is corrected to feel better.

Topic 2: Key Takeaways

If I had to summarize the three most impactful principles I learned, it would be the following.

What Should Help Me Will Hurt Me

If my sorting system isn't working, whatever I did to fight the problem became a part of the problem.

- Internal Helpers—hormones and chemicals the body creates to help.
- External Helpers—medication, supplements, or food.
- Think prevention—think equal sign.

What Goes in Must Come Out

If my body wasn't doing its part in this, I could manually do it myself.

- Avoid forcing Good Guys being grabbed up.
    - Be cautious during times of inflammation.
    - Make manual off-ramps to prevent Helpers from being part of the problem.
- Think protect Good Guys—think equal sign.

Only Give the Body What It Can Handle

Altering my surroundings helped me to control the workload by changing the DISH frequency.

- Baby steps avoids inflammation.
- Inflammation is always a sign something needs to be reprogrammed.
- Think lighten the load—think equal sign.

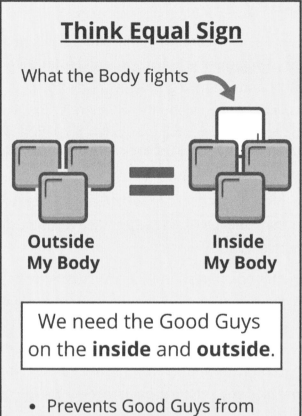

Think Equal Sign

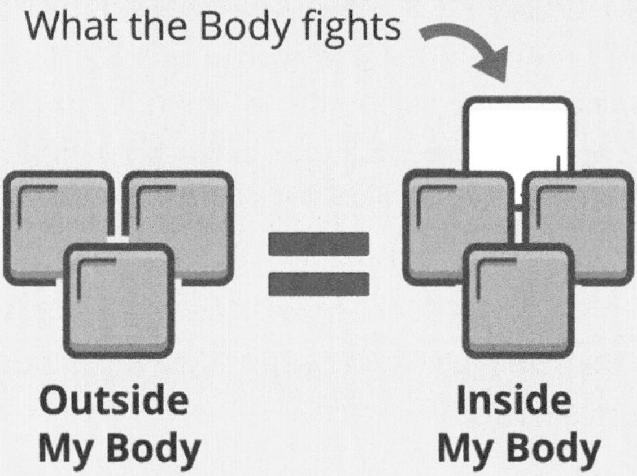

We need the Good Guys on the **inside** and **outside**.

- Prevents Good Guys from being rejected (deficiencies).
- Prevents my body from needing to power down to protect itself (Inflammation).
- Prevents my body from attacking itself (autoimmune disease).

Topic 3: Make Your Health Your Number One Priority

Our bodies were meant to fight Bad Guys and to heal themselves. Something is making this more difficult for some of us. I think understanding DISH is a way for us to remove this *something* problem from the equation. If I am wrong and all the things I have seen happen to me are just made up in my head, then I'm just a crazy old lady who has gone off her rocker. Steer clear of me. But I ask you, if I know some people will think this of me AND **I am writing this book anyway**... don't you think maybe I think what I've figured out is pretty important to share?

I know this does not sound like a fun hobby by any stretch of the imagination. But if I didn't have my health, no matter how fun other hobbies were, it didn't matter. I couldn't physically do them. I wanted to be at least trying to do something about my situation in hopes of someday being able to practice my other hobbies again. So, for now, any spare time I had, I was looking for answers in unusual places. I was looking for patterns and connections and learning. So much learning.

A famous Albert Einstein quote is, "The definition of insanity is doing the same thing over and over again and expecting different results." I was doing everything I was taught to do about healthful living, but it wasn't working. I decided I needed to start over. So, I did, but backwards.

I have now shared with you all the information I have learned so far. I know this is only the tip of the iceberg. I'm going to keep going with this. I have pretty much told you your shoe MIGHT be untied. You can look, or not, to see if it is true.

You can then tie your shoelace and go faster or leave it and trip. You might still get where you are going, just at a slower pace. Or you might trip and have a hard time standing up again. Every person's health journey is unique. That is why each person should be ultimately responsible for their own health.

If at some point you are accused of obsessing over your health, I'd like you to think about two things. If you were an elite athlete and spent that much time learning how to cut two seconds off your time for some event, you wouldn't be considered strange. How much more so wanting to get your health back? The problem is that most of us aren't elite athletes and most of us have to make a living in other ways. This is why health is pushed back to hobby.

The other thing is, if you are like me at all, sometimes I have to talk out loud in order to think. The process of articulating and sharing helped me to process. So, to prevent it from driving my loved ones away, I started journaling. I wrote it down instead of talking their ears off. I encourage you to do the same. Write it down. It will help the process and the patterns to reveal themselves.

Your doctor cares about you. But at the end of the day, if the doctor is a good doctor, for his or her own health she needed to close the book on the patients she had seen for the day. For her own health, she couldn't take her work home with her. You are the one who has to leave the office and live with your body from day to day. It is up to you. Sometimes that is not a good thing to hear.

Because of that, I had to take an active role in my health. And yes, some doctors don't like it when you do this because they think you are trying to tell them how to do their job. That isn't the case. Remember people skills and remember the Venn diagram. Just strive to make the overlap as large as possible. The more they know about you, the more they can help.

Action Steps Summary

I hope you are able to grasp the idea that maybe the reason we can't find what is wrong with us sometimes is because IT IS INVISIBLE. This possible invisible system has many working parts. Working parts that need to come together to work.

- Start off protecting myself.
  - Determine where the body is deficient.
  - What organs are having challenges?
  - What nutrient is in common for them?
  - Hold those nutrients somewhere on me until my body was no longer working on them.
- If that didn't work, I would treat it like a heterogeneous batch.
  - I would do a batch neutralizing session.
  - I would control my environment so I could focus on a smaller batch (triangle) before moving forward.
- If still not working, I would advance to a homogeneous batch.
  - This is when I would search for the Bad Guy.
  - Look for common ground of a resemblance batch.
  - Mixing may have occurred, causing a Good Guy and a Bad Guy to be stuck together.
  - Do the method for homogeneous batches.
- If still not working, look for Mimickers.

  - Some are known already.
  - Some are not.
- Last resort, search for nesting batches.
- So far, every time, one of these methods worked for me.

In this book I have not told you what to take or what to include in your batches. This may frustrate some of you. I am sorry. I can only share with you what I know. I know how this system works. This system is like a cooking pot. I have given you this cooking pot. You need to talk to a health professional to find out what ingredients to put in this pot or whether or not to even use the pot I have given you.

In Closing

Thank you for reading this book through to the end. I am pretty sure I shared with you some information that has you asking questions. I hope so. Run with those questions! Don't take my word for it. I wouldn't. When my world was first rocked for alternative approaches to correcting health challenges, I questioned everything! I would have a thirty-minute appointment every week for a couple of months in the beginning of this health journey. A week was not much time. I would spend hours researching and investigating what she told me. I wanted to know why it was possible what she suggested would work. I also wanted the answer to where I stood on the new information before going to my next already scheduled appointment. I may not have agreed with why she thought what she suggested worked, but maybe there was another possible why for it to work. I always seemed to find one.

"It is impossible for a man 'to learn what he thinks he already knows.'" —Epictetus

As you do your searching and questioning, try to avoid assuming anything. I know great gains have been made by the compounded knowledge of so many scientists before us, but… maybe we don't know what we don't know.

The Big Five of healthy living works for most people, I think, because it keeps the DISH working. But if the wrong programming infiltrated the system, it needs to be rebooted. This is a way I found to correct this information. It worked for me. I want to share it with you. By sharing it with you, I am NOT suggesting you do this. I am just sharing. Sharing something I found fascinating and unbelievable.

Is it safe? I don't know. I am not a doctor. I am just someone who was drowning in the middle of a very turbulent ocean. I found a life raft to jump onto until a rescue boat showed up. Right now, the raft is on very rough waters, but it is keeping me afloat. That is good enough for me.

More Information

"What the mind

doesn't understand,

it worships or fears."

—Alice Walker

GLOSSARY

AFTER: Acronym for Altering Fields to Enable Recovery. The process of manipulating my immediate surroundings with physical objects or colors to manually make an artificial DISH.

Asymptomatic: Having a condition but showing no signs of having the condition.

Attackers: A special group of Good Guys the body makes in order to confront Bad Guys and remove them.

Bad Guy: Anything that is in the body that shouldn't be there. Some refer to this as toxins, but since that word means different things to different people, I prefer to use a unique word.

Batch Neutralizing Session: This is when I sit and slowly introduce into my energy field parts of my environment, essential oils, remedies, food, supplements, and anything else associated with the batch.

Batches: This is a group of Bad Guys or Bad and Good Guys mixed together.

Binders: It is a supplement that attempts to absorb the Bad Guys that have been activated so the body doesn't have to reabsorb them and process them out.

Bridge: The term used when talking about how many items I am holding in order to make the most amount of exit ramps possible.

Byproduct: What is left when a Bad Guy is destroyed.

Canceled Batch: Something was missing from the batch so the batch would need to start over if something was eaten.

Chronic Inflammation: Inflammation that has been going on for a long time.

Cleanser: It is a supplement that attempts to clean up the organs that are trying to remove the Bad Guys so they can do a better job.

Complete Batch: All Bad Guys that needed to be included were included. Progress is made.

Cycles: Passing through a complete meridian clock.

Cycling a Batch: Periodically addressing one item in the batch at a time because the body is too weak to do them all at once because the main target is missing.

DISH: Acronym for Defensive Individual Shield Hypothesis. I use interchangeably with "shield." I am referring to the energy field that my body is creating.

Drop: When a Kingpin is neutralized, there will be a surge of work for the organs to process out.

Dump: When a Bad Guy has been neutralized from a Good Guy resulting in the need to replenish the Good Guy by front loading.

Energy: The ability to do work.

Exposure Batch: I was exposed to the items at the same time. For example: Styrofoam and coffee.

Feingold Diet: The short answer is a diet absent of additives or preservatives.

Front Loading: Taking nutritional supplements (not necessarily full doses) in close proximity over a short period of time to replenish what has been dumped from the body.

Gatekeeper: Another word I use for "target" when holding it enabled me to work on everything else under it in the batch.

Good Guys: Something that is supposed to be in the body.

Growing a Batch: This is a process of adding in more Bad Guys—in groups or one at a time—to the already existing target Bad Guy.

Helper: A vitamin, mineral, food, supplement, medication, or the like that I was using to improve my health.

Heterogeneous Batch: A batch that consists of a group of Bad Guys that can be distinguished one from another.

Hit: When I feel fine and will suddenly feel very ill. Changing what I am holding and not maintaining the same environment for two hours corrects the symptoms. It is usually a sign of a Mimicker or homogeneous batch being corrected.

Hold or holding: This is just having the Bad Guy within my energy field. The distance can vary from skin contact on a specific spot to being a few inches from my body. (Usually.)

Homeopathy: The practice of medicine that believes like cures like and the body wants to heal itself.

Homogeneous Batch: A batch unable to become smaller by separating the Bad Guys from each other. The Bad Guys have become *changed* to where they can only leave as a single unit.

Identify: This is when the Bad Guy first appears on the scene. I needed my body to recognize what it was.

Incomplete Batch: One or more Bad Guys are missing that needed to be included in order for the batch to proceed.

Inflammation: The body's protective reaction to a Bad Guy.

Kingpin: This is a significant target that acts as a Mimicker. It holds several batches together.

Layers: 1.) The different Bad Guys stacked on a meridian.

2.) The various degrees the body goes through while using the AFTER protocol. It consists of the Protection Mode, Train the Body, Target the Bad Guy, and Remove the Kingpin.

Lipids: They help provide energy, produce hormones, aid in digestion and absorption of food, and help the nervous system with signaling.

Mass: The amount of matter that makes up an object.

Meridian: It is a road energy travels on through the body to go to specific organs.

Meridian Clock: The meridians in the body follow a regular schedule in a regular order every day. Each meridian is designated a two-hour time slot.

Metabolic: The adjective used when referring to metabolism.

Metabolism: It refers to the chemical process of the body changing the food and drink we consume into the energy we need for our bodies to function properly. Often low metabolism is attributed to weight gain.

Mimicker: A Bad Guy replicating an essential nutrient or hormone the body needs.

Mimicker Batch: A batch formed around a Mimicker where a Bad Guy is mistakenly identified as a Good Guy.

Nesting: A batch that has one of the Bad Guys as a batch as well.

Neutral Environment: An area where I was the strongest energy field around and the environment did not change by other objects or people entering or exiting my immediate area.

Neutralize: This is when an individual Bad Guy or *a stuck group* (homogeneous batch) has been singled out from the rest of the Bad Guys in the batch. The body has targeted it to where it will become strong enough to now fight it, by itself.

On Top: This is when the same Bad Guy is at the surface of each part of the body being affected.

Organ Section on Meridian Clock: The two-hour section of time that corresponds to a particular organ or groups of organs.

Pecking Order: The order procedures need to be done in.

pH Level: A range for measuring acidity based on 0 being the most acidic and 14 being the basest. 7 would be neutral—too base can burn just as easily as too acidic.

Pillars: This is the name I gave the areas the body consisted of. It refers to the 12 meridians, the governing vessel, the conception vessel, the qi meridian, the nervous system, and corresponding groups of organs. Not all pillars are involved every time.

POOP: Product of other product. Sometimes the Byproduct was so harmful to my body that I needed to treat it as a Bad Guy as well.

Proximity Batch: A Good Guy became attached to the Bad Guy just because they were in the same area of the body. Helpers (Good Guys or medication) would become attached to the organ it was targeting.

Pusher: It is a supplement that attempts to push the Bad Guys out of your body.

Release: This is when the Bad Guy is on top of all the pillars. Once this happens, the body is able to neutralize this individual Bad Guy everywhere the body is being affected. The individual Bad Guy becomes a nonissue for the body.

Remove: This released individual Bad Guy is now just hanging out and waiting for the Bad Guys that are connected to him to also be released. Once they are all released, they can then be removed from the body.

Resemblance Batch: The items were like each other. For example: kerosene and gasoline.

Security Guards: Good Guys in the body who decide if the item is supposed to be in the system or not.

Shield: It is the S in the DISH acronym. I use it interchangeably with DISH. I am referring to the energy field that my body is creating.

Shields Down: My DISH is failing to do its two jobs of protecting and sorting.

Shields Up: My DISH is working properly by protecting the body with a tiny little force field giving off a frequency.

Sway Testing: A technique used to muscle test yourself. See Appendix A.

Symptomatic: The patient has a condition with visible signs of the condition.

Target: The Bad Guy being focused on.

Tiers: The difficulty level of the jobs required to keep the shields up. It consists of Prevention Mode, Easy Batches, and Hard Batches.

Top Target: The Bad Guy who is the chief player in an individual batch.

Training Batch: This is a procedure done to train a heterogeneous batch to recognize the difference between a Good Guy and a Bad Guy when they have become stuck together.

Trigger: An item part of a batch but currently is not included in the batch. If I came into contact with it, the batch would then include it and everything else it is associated with. The challenge here is that it may grow the batch too quickly.

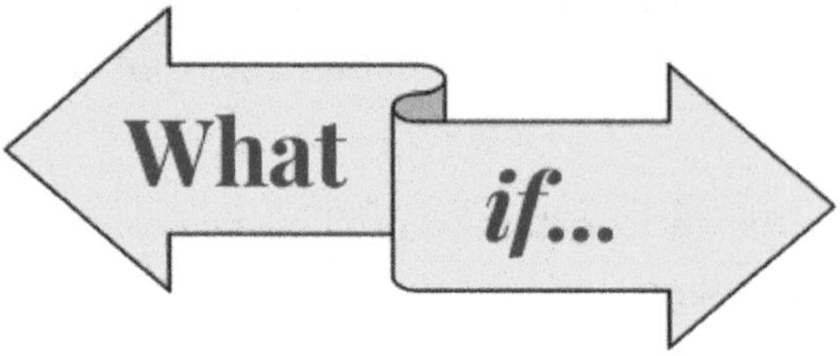

APPENDIX A:

SWAY TESTING/MUSCLE TESTING

This is a partial excerpt from my blog post. It can be found in its entirety at: https://desperatetobewell.com/how-to-sway-test-effectively-get-results/.

How to sway test: Standard Protocol

- Be hydrated.
- Be facing north.
- Sitting or standing is fine.
- Clear my mind.
- Relax.
- Ask the question.
    - A sway forward is yes.
    - A sway backwards is no.

How I Sway Tested: My Protocol

However, for me, it seemed like my conscious mind would always try to be in charge when I did it this way. Through trial and error, I found that by following a slightly different protocol, the answers were more pronounced for me.

1. Take a drink of water.

2. Decide on the question I wanted answered.

3. Deliberately make my conscious mind do something else. It could be something that required little thought. For example, brushing my teeth or peeling carrots. But it had to be focused on something other than the answer I wanted.

4. Then, in the middle of the activity, ask the question. Somehow this helped the subconscious mind to speak up. It kept the conscious mind from overriding the answer by what I wanted the answer to be. (When there is a struggle between the conscious and subconscious mind, the sway is very subtle. (The more "sidetracked" the conscious mind is, the more pronounced the answer is.)

5. Over time, this no longer became a required step. In fact, when I started thinking about what questions to ask, the body would already be swaying the answer.

It is a learned skill:

1. How to practice
    - **a.** Prepare myself.
    - **b.** Recognizing a "yes" answer tends to be easier.
    - **c.** Start with what I do know: Pointer>> Stick with looking at a cup or a glass and saying what they are.
    - **d.** Be patient.
2. Trouble-shooting
    - **a.** Be hydrated.
    - **b.** Get on my knees: This will change the fulcrum location to make the answer more pronounced.
    - **c.** Be more specific in my question.

3. Bedridden: I can still do the sway test. Instead of practicing with yes answers, I will want to practice with no answers. It is easier to feel a "no" than a "yes." I will be pushed into the bed with *no*. The *yes* answer may just be no push at all if I was very quick. Eventually, it may become a head nod, then a shoulder raise as my strength returned.

When it still doesn't seem to be working:

Sometimes the body will not sway at all. Other times it might sway both ways. I have learned that these are neither yeses or noes but "it depends."

How I Say It Matters:

1. Only ask questions with one clear interpretation of the question.

2. Avoid negative words like *not* or *can't*. It will not understand *not*, and *can't* will be interpreted as *can*.

3. Remember the magic words.

   a. **With:** Needs to be combined with something.
   b. **And:** Something else also needed to be done either before, during, or afterwards.

4. And if all else failed. Ask: Can I get a "yes" right now? If no, wait and try again later or have someone else test for me.

Examples:

- Hold this item and then I will be able to take this supplement.
- Yes, I can eat this, but first take this vitamin and wait ten minutes.
- No, the body is overburdened and I need to wait, then it will be safe.
- Yes, but not right now. Something else has to happen first.
- Yes, but away from all electricity.
- Take this supplement, and then take the next one.

In a way, it is like dealing with a newborn. The baby is crying because she is trying to communicate something to me. A type of intuition of understanding the communication process between the conscious and subconscious mind. To get to the source of what the body needs is what we are aiming for.

APPENDIX B:

BASIC SCIENCE REVIEW

Mass & Energy: In this equation, the letters represent the following:

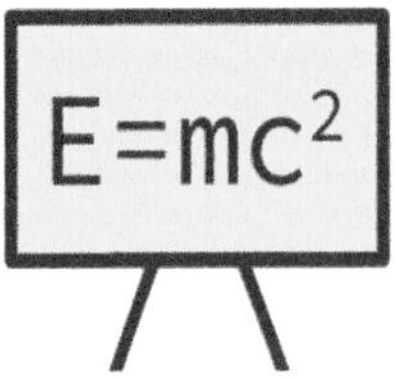

E = Energy M = Mass C = Speed of Light

What does this infamous equation Albert Einstein came up with actually mean?

$E = mc^2$: This equation is German-born physicist Albert Einstein's theory of special relativity. It expresses the fact that mass and energy are the same physical entity and can be changed into each other.[86]

pH Levels: Most people know acid burns. What most people don't know is that base burns just as much. The farther away from neutral you get, the more potential of *being harmed*.

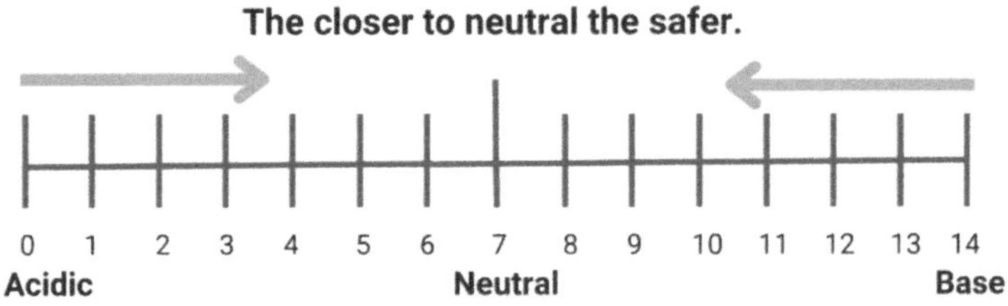

[86] Perkowitz, Sidney. "E=mc^2." Britannica. Last accessed 27 March 2023. https://www.britannica.com/science/E-mc2-equation.

Radioactivity: Everything is made up of atoms. An atom contains protons, neutrons, and electrons. The number of protons determines what element the atom is.

- Excess neutrons cause the atom to be heavier than normal.
- This heaviness is what makes the atom become an isotope.
- Isotopes are stable and unstable (radioactive).

For example, Strontium-90 (Bad Guy) and strontium (Good Guy) are both strontium. Strontium has the elemental number of 38. The 90 at the end of strontium-90 tells us there is an excess of 52 neutrons. These extra neutrons undergo radioactive decay, making this strontium isotope radioactive.[87]

Venn Diagram: A way of sorting items into groups to look at what is shared between the groups. :

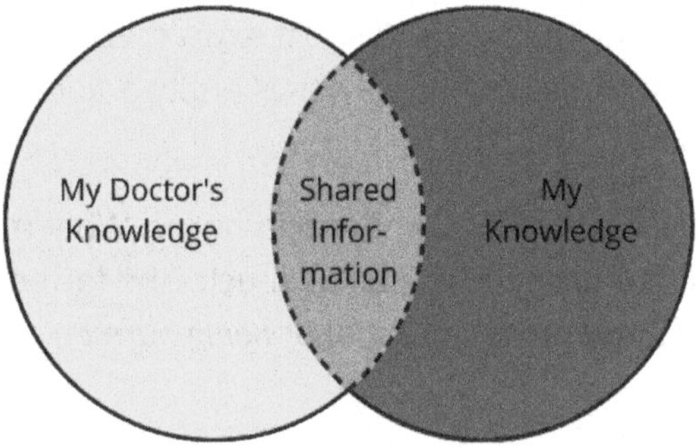

I think waves canceling each other is the missing piece we have been looking for.

---

[87] Office of Science. "DOE Explains... Isotopes." Energy Gov—Office of Science. Last accessed 28 March 2023. https://www.energy.gov/science/doe-explainsisotopes.

Waves: Just as it is difficult to wrap my head around the idea that everything I am looking at on my computer screen is a result of nothing but a bunch of zeros and ones, I choose to believe this is the case rather than to try to completely understand how the different parts of waves work together.

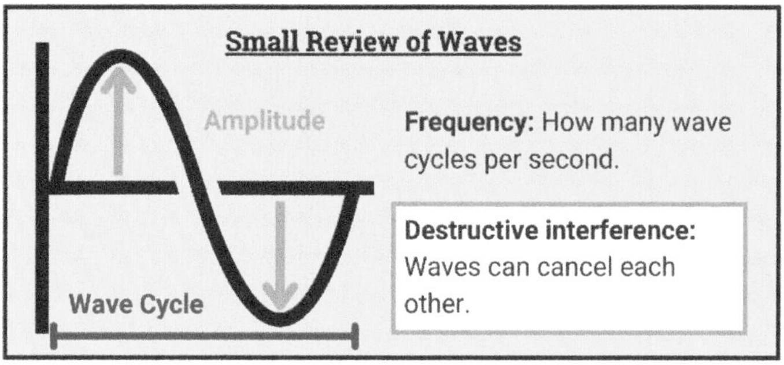

It is easy to get caught up in the details of what makes a wave. If you don't understand it, that is okay. The main point is... waves can cancel each other. I think the label for the lesson from Ohio State University says it all. [88]

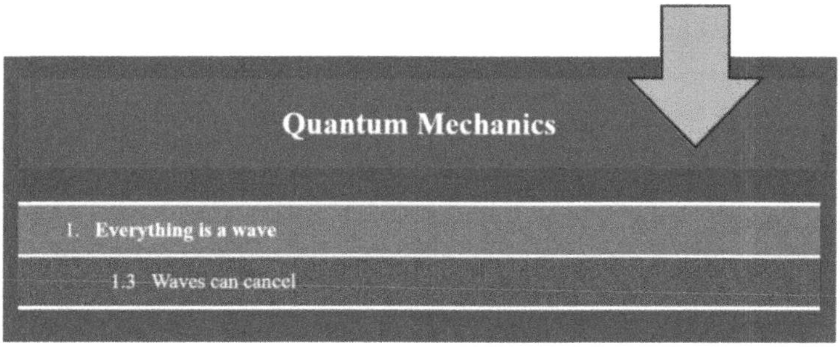

[88] Ohio State University. "Quantum Mechanics." Ohio State University. Last accessed 27 March 2023. https://www.asc.ohio-state.edu/mathur.16/quantummechanics27-11-17/qm1.3/qm1.3.html.

APPENDIX C:

BOOKS WHERE MY RETHINKING BEGAN

This book would not have been possible without first expanding my mind with the following publications. Thank you, authors, for writing them.

1. *A small amount mattered: Living Gluten Free for Dummies* by Danna Korn.

2. *The answer could be simple: The Body's Many Cries for Water* by F. Batmanghelidj, MD.

3. *It's all about energy: NAET: Allergy Book* by Devi S. Nambudripad, MD.

4. *The mind can be trained: The Gift of Dyslexia* by Ronald D. Davis and Eldon M. Braun.

5. *The body remembers everything: The Emotion Code* by Dr. Bradley Nelson.

I have combined all I learned from these books & countless hours of internet research to come up with what I have learned and written in this book.

APPENDIX D:

MEET THE AUTHOR

Cyndi earned her Bachelor of Science degree in 1991. She married Ron in 1992, served a short term as a commissioned Air Traffic Control officer in the Air Force, then became a stay-at-home mom.

Cyndi's parents became pregnant with her at Camp Lejeune. It would be later discovered this Marine base had contaminated water containing many harmful components, including strontium-90 and benzene at levels ranging from 240 to 3,400 times higher than what is permitted by safety standards. In Cyndi's early years, she lived in New Zealand and Turkey. She remained a military dependent until her dad retired when she was in eighth grade.

Find her at desperatetobewell.com (blog), cyndiwhatif.com (author site), or healthbackwards.com (book site).

More Books to Come

Health Backwards: The Journal

- A guide for your medical journey.
- Packed with information and questions to use to search for answers.
- It is not medical advice, but a medical tool to help make quicker progress.

Health Backwards Part Two: How I Implemented AFTER

- A detailed look at how I did the procedures I have shared in this book.
- It builds off Health Backwards.

ACKNOWLEDGMENTS

First of all, I would like to thank my writing professor. She believed I should be a writer when I refused to believe it myself. Her belief in me those thirty-plus years ago gave me enough courage to tackle this task of writing a book. I finally took your advice and did it! I found a purpose big enough to write about. It is not the book you wanted me to write, but maybe, someday, it will spill onto the pages too.

I would like to thank my beta readers. I greatly appreciated your feedback and loved the insight and encouragement you gave me. Without you, I could not have morphed this book into what it is now. It is barely a shell of the first draft. Thank you.

I had several different doctors and types of doctors, but I would like to thank specifically two individuals.

➢ Barbara Leonard, acupuncturist, homeopath, herbalist, friend.

You were there with me when my health was at its worst. You were so patient with my endless questions. If you weren't willing to answer them, I may have just given up and never journeyed down this new road I have found.

➢ Aaron Chapa, ACN

Thank you for being patient with me. I know I was not exactly your *normal* patient. Your willingness to work with me enabled me to clarify my thoughts enough to be able to put them in a book. My desire for you to understand what I was going through is what caused this book to be born.

➢ Abigail, Zach, Josiah, Sam, Sarah, Nathan, and my husband, Ron.

Last but not least, my family. Thank you for helping me through my darkest days, being patient with me in my frustrating days, supporting me in my discovering days, and believing in me during the writing of this book.

Made in the USA
Monee, IL
28 July 2023

39870449R00234